PATIENT by PATIENT

ALSO BY EMILY R. TRANSUE, M.D.

On Call: A Doctor's Days and Nights in Residency

PATIENT by PATIENT

Lessons in Love, Loss,
Hope, and Healing from
a Doctor's Practice

Emily R. Transue, M.D.

 St. Martin's Griffin ✳ New York

www.stmartins.com

Book design by Sarah Maya Gubkin

The Library of Congress has catalogued the hardcover edition as follows:

Transue, Emily R.
    Patient by patient : lessons in love, loss, hope, and healing from a doctor's practice / Emily R. Transue.—1st ed.
        p. cm.
    ISBN-13: 978-0-312-37278-1
    ISBN-10: 0-312-37278-7
    1. Transue, Emily R. 2. Internists—Washington (State)—Seattle—Biography.
3. Physician and patient. 4. Physician-Patient Relations—Personal Narratives.
5. Attitude to Death—Personal Narratives. 6. Family Relations—Personal
Narratives. 7. Physicians, Women—Personal Narratives. I. Title.
    R154.T673 A3 2008
    610.69'6092—dc22
    [B]

                                                                    2008001804

    ISBN-13: 978-0-312-37279-8 (pbk.)
    ISBN-10: 0-312-37279-5 (pbk.)

First St. Martin's Griffin Edition: April 2009

10 9 8 7 6 5 4 3 2 1

AUTHOR'S NOTE

Names and identifying characteristics have been changed to preserve confidentiality.

To Chris Knight, with much love

CONTENTS

ACKNOWLEDGMENTS

I would like to thank: first of all, my wonderful family, many of whom are not represented in these pages. My mother, Harriet Adams; my brother, Kit Transue; and my stepfather, John Straub, who have been supportive beyond words, and who are tremendous sources of inspiration in my work and life. My grandmother, my grandfather, and my father, whom I have tried to honor but whose stories I could not hope to tell adequately. My uncles and aunt, Bill and Virginia and John Transue. Arnold Zwicky, to whom I owe a debt I could never begin to repay.

The people who get me through my workdays: Chris Pepin and Marti Liddell, with special thanks also to Rachel and Clare and Rob Liddell, my beloved professional in-laws. The mentors of my academic and writing careers: Blair Brooks, Doug Paauw, Erika Goldstein, Dawn DeWitt, among others. The many friends who have encouraged me in my writing, most of all Dennis Rivet and Shala Erlich. Judy and Kelly Foss, whose gift of time in a beautiful place enabled me to finish this manuscript. The University of Washington medical students in my writing class, who have been a huge joy and inspiration. The staff who keep my office running—too many to list, but including Bobbi, Christine, Cindy, Danielle, Kearstyn, Lisa, Marissa, Marquessa, Melinda, Nancy, and Tasha.

My agent, Joan Raines, without whose encouragement this book would have never come into existence. Diane Reverand, Dana Grossman and the staff of *Dartmouth Medicine*, Roxanne Young at *JAMA*, and Nell Casey at *Self* for their support and encouragement and good editing. Sheila Curry Oakes and everyone at St. Martin's Press for supporting the book and helping me make it so much better.

Robert Coles, who offered kind words on top of his incredibly inspiring example.

Almost last but certainly not least, Chris Knight, who has kept me going through all the stages of creating this book, and through the experiences that went into it.

Finally, I would like to thank my patients, both those who are in this book and those who are not. Thank you for sharing your lives and stories, and for teaching me so much about doctoring and about life.

BEGINNINGS

1. ANOTHER BEGINNING

As I pressed my new parking sticker carefully onto my windshield, I paused to consider the enormity of what the small sliver of plastic represented. At the age of twenty-nine, with twenty-four continuous years of education under my belt, I was about to begin what could be called my first real job. My new business card burned in my pocket: "Emily R. Transue, MD, General Internal Medicine." I was starting practice as a primary care physician.

With a laugh, I thought back to the day I'd decided to go to medical school. It was early in my senior year in college; I'd been a biology major, scrambling for a new career path after realizing I didn't want to spend my life at a lab bench. I'd done Parkinson's research with primates, and reasoned that if monkeys were interesting, people must be even more so. I called my grandparents to announce my momentous decision.

"But we hate doctors," my grandmother protested.

Through all my years of medical training, whenever a physician amputated the wrong leg, administered the wrong medication, or made some other terrible mistake, my grandmother would send me a news clipping. I was never sure if these were warnings about what might occur if I applied myself inadequately, or simply further evidence for the argument that physicians were an untrustworthy lot. During my second year of medical school, she called to tell me that my grandfather had developed atrial fibrillation, an irregular heart rhythm. It's usually treated with blood thinners, to reduce the risk of a clot forming in the heart and traveling to the brain, and cardioversion, a brief electrical shock to restore the heart rhythm. "They're giving your grandfather rat poison," my grandmother declared. Rat poison is made from warfarin, the same compound used medicinally to thin blood. "Then they're going to electrocute him."

I had to admit that these were precisely the kinds of barbaric things that people in my chosen profession did.

Still, here I was. Absurdly, the parking sticker brought home what my contract, my application for hospital privileges, the ordering of office letterhead and exam room supplies, and all the other events of the past weeks had not. In the eight years since I had started medical school, everything I had done had been temporary. Student clerkships lasted four to eight weeks, residency rotations a month. My year as a chief resident, teaching and helping run the program I had finished the year before, was the longest I had spent in any single role, and even that was clearly defined as transient; my successor was chosen before I'd even started. In all that time I had hung temporary parking placards from my rearview mirror. The sticky teal rectangle on my front window seemed to symbolize the end to transience and the unfamiliar permanence I was entering. After eight years of working toward this role, I had arrived.

A few weeks before, the ink barely dry on my employment contract, I had signed another sheaf of papers, buying a house with my sweetheart, also a doctor starting his first job. Our possessions were still in boxes, the wonder of owning a piece of land and the home that sat on it still fresh. As I finished affixing the parking sticker and walked into the angular brick and glass building of the clinic, I was bursting with the richness and strangeness of my new life. I had a house, a job, a piano, two cats, a life partner. I was a long way from Ohio, where I grew up, and from New Hampshire, where I went to medical school. I was far from my family. My brother was doing computer work in Boston; my mother had left her college professor position in Ohio to go to law school in Washington, D.C. Most acutely, I felt my distance from the ones who weren't well: my father, who recently had moved into a nursing home in California, and his parents—the ones who hated doctors—who were close to ninety but still living independently in Pennsylvania in the house where my grandfather grew up.

Nonetheless, I had laid down my roots here, in Seattle. I could feel them in the earth under the maple tree in my new front yard, and even in the glue of the parking sticker. I was about to walk into the clinic and begin to grow roots of another kind, putting on my white coat and meeting strangers who would become my patients, as I grew into my role as their doctor.

I felt the joint tug of responsibility to the people I loved and to the patients I would begin caring for today. I had finished the hard years of residency, the hundred-hour weeks and thirty-six-hour shifts, the drama of the hospital and the emergency room. I had seen a lot of people die or nearly die in those years, and I thought I knew plenty about grief and loss and healing. I little imagined how much more and how differently I would learn in the coming years. Much of this would come from the patients I would care for, not just in the episodic crises of the hospital but in the slower, richer arc of sickness and health that a primary care doctor sees. In parallel, my first years in practice would be tumultuous ones for the people in the world I loved most, and I would see more than I ever had of medicine from the other side.

I could only begin to glimpse all this, as the sliding doors opened to admit me to the cool, quiet air of the clinic. My heart sped with a mix of anxiety and excitement as I stepped inside, savoring the newness, and looking forward to a time when I could savor familiarity instead.

2. FIRST DAYS

The first patient I saw, that first September morning, was a young woman with sciatic back pain. "I bent over to pick up a pile of books and there was this sudden, terrible pain in my back. It shoots down my leg all the way to my foot."

She was uncomfortable, but not in crisis. It was a simple problem; a medical student would have known what to do. I gave her medication to reduce the inflammation and to quiet her pain. I told her which activities she should and shouldn't do, when to expect the pain to get better, and when to call me if it didn't. The interaction went just fine, but I don't know that I had ever been as nervous managing a heart attack or massive stroke as I was with that young woman's sore back. I schooled my voice carefully to keep it from trembling. I double-checked the details of the prescriptions I had written, which looked oddly unfamiliar on the fresh pad printed with my name. The question kept popping into my mind: What if what I'm telling her isn't right? I had to keep reminding myself that it was, that I *did* know how to do this. I'd had similar conversations many times in training, but afterward I had always gone to present my findings to my supervisor, gotten advice or a stamp of approval. From here on, though I could and often would ask advice of my colleagues, there would be nobody above me. I was on my own. With that first patient, that fact in itself was terrifying.

My second patient had a urinary tract infection, and was a little easier. The third was in for a physical exam, and soon I was so caught up in learning about her history and her concerns that I didn't think to be nervous. By the end of the day the fact that I didn't have to run things by anyone didn't seem so strange. By the end of the first week I had stopped thinking about it.

My clinic is a large, doctor-owned group, which represents almost all the medical specialties. I chose it partly for this, knowing I would have colleagues to talk to, to ask questions of, to learn from. I had completed four years of residency training on top of the four years of medical school. I had passed my specialty boards in Internal Medicine. "It's like being a pediatrician for adults," I explained to friends who didn't know what an internist was. "No kids, no OB, no surgery, but pretty much everything else." I had the tools I needed, but there was lots of practical, day-to-day knowledge I had yet to learn. They call it "practice" for a reason, I reminded myself.

The clinic building was yellow brick and glass, with several wings built at different times. Medical buildings, ever-expanding according to need, have always reminded me of swallows' nests, the structures of one era tacked onto those of the age before. My office was on the second floor in the older part of the building, its window looking out onto a quiet street and the steeple of a nearby church. I had my own medical assistant and would soon hire a receptionist (the title would later change to "patient service representative," roles shifting and evolving like the building, like medicine itself). I had two examination rooms, small and neat but a little dark. After years of rotating through rooms in the resident clinic, I realized to my great delight that these rooms were mine to set up as I chose. I replaced the ugly, industrial mirror in each room with a pretty, modern one, and added a floor lamp. Suddenly the rooms seemed brighter and the note of dinginess was gone. I began to fill the walls with photographs, the plain yellow paint giving way to scenes of mountains and wildflowers. I put fuzzy covers on the cold metal stirrups of my exam tables. After a few weeks I realized that the rooms no longer felt like just exam rooms: they felt like *my* exam rooms. It was a subtle difference but a transforming one.

As I rearranged and settled into my office and my newly bought house, I felt that I was building a home of sorts in both spaces. My new life was beginning to take shape.

The saving grace of starting practice was that I had friends from residency going through the same thing. Periodically we would gather to debrief about the strangeness of this new world.

"I saw this guy in coverage today that I wanted to steal from his regular doctor."

"Steal?"

"To have him come to me for primary care. You know? He was just such a nice guy, we had a great chat. If all your patients were that nice, it'd be the perfect job."

I laughed. "I've had people like that. You think, I would smile every time I saw you were coming in." I thought of a sweet seventy-year-old I had seen that day with nosebleeds, anxious to have them stop before she went to Europe with her son. We'd talked about my trips to Europe with my mother, about Italy, about grown children traveling with their mothers. She'd smiled, and as she was leaving she said shyly, "You're nice—" In that moment all the years of work I'd done to get to this job felt worth it.

"It's so weird having such an open schedule. We didn't have this much time for new patients when we were residents, even."

"I know. It's neat, you feel like you really have time to talk."

"Sure. But I find myself doing these ridiculous things, just because I have the time. I feel like I need to do all the health care that people haven't had in the last five years. Someone comes in for sinusitis and I have an empty schedule so suddenly I'm reviewing their whole family history and giving them a tetanus shot and trying to check their prostate. They're like, 'I just wanted antibiotics!'"

I nodded. "I did a Pap smear yesterday on someone who came in with an earache."

He giggled. "Poor people. . . ."

"It's kind of like an assault."

" 'Leave me alone! I felt bad enough when I came in here.' "

———

Meantime, I was learning a new kind of medicine. Residency had trained me brilliantly to think of things to worry about; I was not so adept at deciding which of those I needed to take seriously. Much of my training had been in the hospital, where we were dealing with urgent issues and often doing lots of tests at once. The rhythm of clinic medicine was different; few problems were emergencies, and it was usually better to approach the evaluation one step at a time. Furthermore, in contrast to the hospital where almost everyone had something seriously wrong, in clinic half the challenge was figuring out who wasn't sick. The hardest part was often reassuring people that their bodies just needed time to heal on their own.

Though the approach was different, the learning curve was as steep as it had been in residency, those packed years of specialty training after medical school. A lot of the time I felt like I had then: excited, and exhausted, and thrilled to be finally doing something that I'd been training for so long. I wasn't yet efficient at clinic medicine, so the difference between a too-quiet schedule and a too-busy one was only a few patients. I could turn on a dime from feeling restless to feeling overwhelmed. My practice grew quickly, though, and my skills grew with it. I was startled to realize one afternoon that I had comfortably seen more patients in half a day than I had in my entire first week.

Some weeks after that first day, a young woman who looked vaguely familiar came in to have a physical exam. She smiled brightly and told me that her back pain had gone away just when I had said it would. Glancing down at her chart, I realized that she had been my very first patient from my very first day. It seemed much longer ago than it was; I couldn't imagine having been quite so nervous over a simple problem just a month or two earlier. She looked around the room and admired a photograph of a rose from my front yard.

"Looks like you've settled in," she said.

"I have."

3. CODING AND COMPLIANCE

Seeing patients was easy to get used to, but the financial and administrative side of medicine was considerably more challenging. During my first week I had a long and baffling meeting with the people from a department I had never previously heard of: Coding and Compliance. The Coding and Compliance staff had the unenviable task of teaching me in a few hours how to bill for the work I do. This had barely been addressed in my four years of post-graduate specialty training, much less in medical school. I'd had eight years of medical training, and nobody had acknowledged that this was a business as well as a calling.

The medical billing process is based on codes that are marked down for each visit. There's one type of code for the visit itself, which depends on the visit's length and complexity. There are also codes for procedures: Everything from heart surgery to giving a shot has a distinct code. Each of these is then linked to a separate diagnosis code—what the visit or the procedure was for. This seemed simple enough. But when the Coding and Compliance specialists—Karen and Linda—started talking, nothing they said made sense. I flashed back to a time when I tried to speak French with someone who was Belgian; the words sounded right, but no actual communication occurred. I wondered if, as on that earlier occasion, it would be better to use mimes and hand gestures.

Karen began. "You've got your basics, your E and M's and your preventatives." I took a breath to ask what these were, but she was already continuing. Somewhere I could remember having heard "E and M" before. Random paired letters flashed through my mind—A&P grocery stores, A&W Root Beer, B&O railroad—wait, I had it! "E and M" was "Evaluation and Management," the code for a visit about a problem. I struggled to catch up to what Karen had been saying in the meantime. "Remember that news are different than follow-ups, although if they've been seen by someone else in the clinic in three years they're not a new, unless it wasn't in your specialty. Remember if it's a consult you have to code a 902 series instead of a 992 series. You have to dictate the referring practitioner or it's not a 902. Remember to differentiate a consultation from a referral, although that won't affect you so much, you're a primary care."

What's the difference between a consultation and a referral? I wondered, but her tone suggested I should have learned this on my grandmother's knee, and I was afraid to ask. Then I thought: I'm "a primary care"? I've been through eight years of training, I've been in practice for two days and I already lost the "doctor" from my title?

I wrote down "902/992" on my notepad and hoped it would mean something to me later.

"You can use the V codes, but remember they're not always reimbursed."

"V codes?" I said weakly.

Karen nodded but didn't elaborate. "And when you've got an eight or a nine hundred then you need to remember your E code; nobody likes it but it's important or the claim will get denied."

"Excuse me?"

"Well, they won't pay for anything if they think maybe someone else should be paying it. L and I, or something."

L and I, Labor and Industries! I was thrilled to finally recognize an acronym.

"I'm sorry, you lost me there again. Eight or nine hundred? E?"

Linda sighed as if I were a particularly truculent child. "Eight or nine hundred codes are things like injuries and accidents. E's are circumstances, locations, and causes. Someone has a broken arm, you have to code an E for how it happened—motor vehicle accident, fall—or else it doesn't get paid. Or if it was at home, you code that, versus if it's at work, and then it would go to L and I."

I wrote down, "8-900, E." I was starting to feel a little nauseated.

"But remember the 800 or 900 has to be first, the E is always a secondary code."

"E secondary," I wrote down.

Through most of the process of orienting to the clinic I'd been excited, albeit nervous. Yes, there was a lot to learn, and yes, this would be different from being a resident; but this was it, it was real, it was what I'd been working toward all these years. By the end of the Coding and Compliance lecture I was a quivering wreck. "I can't do it," I announced when I got home. "This whole thing is a terrible mistake. I just can't do it."

My sweetheart, Chris, was going through the same traumas at his own new job. He soothed me. "Of course you can do it. You've done everything else you needed to do, all along the way. You can do this, too."

The nice thing about complete ignorance is that you have reason to treasure every emerging glimmer of competence. I successfully coded my first sore throats and sinus infections, and felt irrationally triumphant. I started to get excited about coding. I thumbed through the massive coding encyclopedia and discovered codes for obscure problems and even more obscure circumstances. Codes for eyeworms and Familial Mediterranean Fever. Codes for falling off a cliff or out of an airplane.

One day I coded a 917.6: "foreign body—superficial—foot—noninfected" and the accompanying procedure code, CPT 28190: "removal—foreign body—superficial—noninfected—foot."

Linking 917.6 to 28190 meant that I removed a splinter.

I added an E849.0 to note that the splinter was acquired at home, not at a place of work or business. I couldn't decide who would be more stunned: my mother, to know how many 917.6/28190/E849.0s she performed when I was a child; or myself at the time I entered medical school, if I had known this was how I would be spending my time and energy.

Luckily my residency friends, also entering practice, were going through the same process. An e-mail arrived from a friend entitled, "Coding seminar."

"911.0: Abrasion, superficial, trunk [includes penis].

"E918: Caught between two objects."

At the end he added: "Really they should put warning signs on zippers."

Despite my flights of coding fancy, I still had trouble with the basics. Reluctantly, I dialed the Coding and Compliance number.

"I have a couple of questions—"

"We can come down."

Linda and Karen arrived with remarkable alacrity, smiling cheerily. They were very pleasant, and very bright; they just didn't speak the same language I did.

They sat down across the desk from me. I'd already figured out that the process would go better if I had a clear question, so I started briskly.

"I'm trying to figure out this whole thing with the preventative exams," I said. "I understand that there's a distinction in billing between a preventative visit and a treatment visit. But I'm confused about what to do when there are elements of both."

"You shouldn't do both in the same visit."

"I understand that ideally they'll be separate. But I can't tell someone, 'I know you've taken the day off from work to come here and see your doctor, but three of the items on your list are preventative and two are nonpreventative, so you'll just have to come back another day.'"

"I know the doctors don't like it," Karen said severely. "But that's the way the system is."

I tried to explain. "The doctors don't like it because it doesn't fit with the way we think. People come in with questions, and we try to address them. These distinctions seem artificial. I'm trying to understand them so I can work with them."

Linda sighed and shifted uncomfortably in her chair.

"Well, there is one thing you can do. If you really have to do both in one visit, you can do a dot-two-five."

"A what?"

"You can code it as preventative and then do a dot-two-five modifier on an E and M." I had confirmed that "E and M" meant "Evaluation and Management," so I didn't have to embarrass myself by asking this.

Karen looked at Linda in alarm, as if she were divulging state secrets.

"What's that?"

"It's an extra code you can put behind the preventative code, and then you can bill an E and M for the same visit. Like, if at the end of a physical somebody suddenly had chest pain and then you evaluated them for that."

"So I can do both!"

"Yes," said Linda.

"But," said Karen.

"But what?"

"But most insurances don't take dot-two-five modifiers."

"So what happens if I try to code one?"

"Well, it's legal, you won't have committed insurance fraud. But they'll just pay for one of the two; usually they pick the cheaper one."

"So I can bill for both if I do both, I just won't get paid."

"Yes."

"Great."

There was a long pause, while I rubbed my throbbing temples.

"Okay. Let me think about all that for a bit." Then again, I thought, I could save myself a lot of headaches and just open a coffee shop instead. There are no dot-two-five modifiers for coffee.

"My other question is simpler. I'm trying to figure out how to bill a physical. I had someone complain last week because I billed for a physical and it wasn't covered. She said her insurance said they would cover a Pap."

Karen stepped to the plate. "A Pap smear is covered under the state Women's Health Initiative."

Linda added, "And a lot of the HMOs will pay for preventative care."

HMO, Health Maintenance Organization, I thought to myself, trying to take comfort in recognizing another acronym.

"A V70.0 is a physical—are you doing the whole thing? Listening to her heart and lungs? Past history, family history? Of course, if she's a return, it's only an update." She's "a return" in the same way that I'm "a primary care," I thought. We all get abbreviated to our billing functions.

"Of course I am. Most of the time in someone young those are pretty simple, but they could turn up something important."

"If you're just doing a Pap you could code a V72.3, gynecological exam with routine cervical Pap."

"So I should code that instead of a V70.0, physical exam?"

"No, V70.0 is better. A V72.3 assumes you're just swabbing her cervix and not doing anything else. There's less compensation." I'd noticed that the word "compensation" was used instead of "payment," as though money changed hands as a kind of apology for our inconvenience.

"But will the insurance pay for a V70.0? Is that covered under the—" I searched for the term. "The Women's Health Initiative?"

"Not necessarily," Linda said. "Some insurances cover it, some don't."

"Which ones?"

"It's always changing."

"So if I code a V72.3, I don't really get paid for the work I did, but if I code a V70.0, I do, but she might get the bill."

Karen nodded.

"Or she might not, and there's no way for me to know?"

She nodded again.

"We're surprised that this confuses people?" I asked.

There was a long silence. Finally I looked down at my watch. "I think it's time for me to get back to the easy part of my job—seeing patients."

Luckily I enjoy seeing patients, and by the end of the day I was cheery again, and ready to tackle the coding labyrinth once more. Just before I left for home I got a text message from another friend just starting practice.

"Did you know there's an ICD-9 code for legal execution?"

"Really?" I wrote back.

"E978 covers lethal injection, death by firing squad, electrocution, beheading, and other means not otherwise specified."

"Thanks," I wrote back. "I'm glad to know how to code what I want to do to the person who designed this system."

4. ADVICE

As a new doctor at my clinic, I was a magnet for advice. Physicians I had never met came up to me to offer gems and pearls of wisdom, things they wished they'd known when they were starting out. They meant well, all of them; but as a cumulative mass the advice became overwhelming. "Don't give anyone narcotics," I was told. In my first days on call I would get dozens of calls from people saying that they just ran out of Percocet, or that the cat ate their codeine or their ex-boyfriend stole their Valium. "There will be people in your office acting out the death scene from *La Boheme* and telling you you're going to burn in hell if you don't give them Oxycontin. Don't fall for it."

"I had one guy who claimed to be on his way to his wedding," one colleague said. "He said he had a kidney stone and he'd had them before and could I just give him some Vicodin to control the pain through the ceremony. And I was writing out the script when I realized that his tux didn't fit. Nobody gets married in a tux that doesn't fit. From there the whole thing unraveled. But I tell you, I was *this* close."

"But some people really do have kidney stones," I said.

"Don't give out anything unless you are holding a positive CT scan."

"I had this nice young woman the other day with kidney stones. She'd had them before—"

He looked at me knowingly. "Let me guess. She was allergic to contrast dye so she couldn't have a scan, or—no—it was under her deductible and she couldn't afford it."

My eyes widened. "There was blood in her urine—"

"People prick their fingers."

"I think she really had them."

"Talk to me in three months."

In three months, she had come back to me four times for narcotic prescriptions. I pushed her harder about getting a scan, or at least obtaining old records documenting her disease—even assuming her story about the stones was real, I didn't want to be missing a diagnosis or treating the wrong thing. She responded with a scathing letter saying that I was hateful and mean and shouldn't be allowed to see patients. Meantime, she'd started calling on the weekends when other docs were on call, with an untrue story about how I'd put her on stronger painkillers than she wanted and asking the on-call doc to call in "something milder." When the prescriptions dried up she left the clinic.

Other advice was about managing calls on nights and weekends. "Send people to the ER," one colleague said. "You get someone calling in the middle of the night and you can't figure out for sure what's going on, just send them in."

"Don't send anyone to the ER unless you absolutely have to," another doc advised. "New docs always think that—worst comes to worst, I'll just send them to the ER—but then you'll be getting calls from the ER docs at two in the morning to say, hey, your patient is fine, or worse yet: they seem okay but they're here so I've decided to admit them, so you'd better come in."

There was advice about managing my staff, my schedule, my office, my colleagues. "Be flexible," some people told me. "Say yes to anything anyone asks you to do, you can always scale back later." "Set firm limits," others said. "Once things spiral out of control you can never get them back in." Some people recommended having a high threshold for referring patients out to specialists, others a low one. Everyone had a horror story from starting practice that they wanted to share. One had gotten so busy so fast he was overwhelmed and ended up being hospitalized with anxiety and depression. Another left her first job because she'd felt ostracized for refusing to work late hours. "Play the game." "Don't be too nice." "You can spoil everything by taking the wrong steps at this stage in your career. It's happened before—it happened to me. It can happen to you."

Then there were the messages sifting in from the insurance companies and from our malpractice insurer. Be efficient, the insurance companies are counting every dollar you spend. Be complete, leave no stone unturned or you'll be susceptible to a lawsuit. One day we had a long meeting about how expensive transcription was and how all the doctors would have to cut down on the length of their dictations. The next day there was a risk-management meeting about how if we didn't document every thought in our heads and every detail and nuance of each conversation with our patients, we were liable to get sued.

"This is crazy!" I complained to Chris. "It can't be done."

"My office had those same two meetings last week," he said.

Every word of advice was well-meant, and undoubtedly they seemed more ominous to me than anyone intended. People were only trying to prevent me from repeating their mistakes. Still, with every hour bringing a new piece of wisdom and each contradicting the last, I was exhausted and confused. The message seemed to be: There is no way to do it right.

Happily, at last, I came to see this as a blessing as well as a curse. If there was no right answer, I couldn't be expected to have one. As the months went by I made some mistakes, and averted some others. There was a balance to be struck, I realized, between cynicism and gullibility, between offering too much and believing too little. There was usually a line of reasonable medical judgment that fell somewhere between spending a fortune eliminating all uncertainty and saving money by accepting too much. There would be pieces of advice I would take and pieces I would leave, and despite everyone's best intentions, I would have to find my own way.

5. HEMATOSPERMIA

Sometimes the struggle to say and do the right thing was more comic than painful. My schedule lists each patient's name, the time of their appointment, and the reason they're coming, which in medical terms is called the "chief complaint." The word "complaint" once seemed odd to me; are we saying that everyone who comes in is a complainer? Couldn't we use something less charged, perhaps "chief concern"? Over time, this term slipped into the invisibility of constant use. One afternoon a "complaint" on the schedule caught my eye: "Blood in semen."

The man's name was familiar but I tried vainly to attach it to a face. I recognized him, however, as soon as I walked in the door. Young, pleasant, very personable. I'd seen him just once before, and that time he admitted that he'd never seen a woman doctor. This is one of those things you wish people hadn't said, or that they'd waited to say until later: *Hey, isn't it funny, but that first time—.* When they say it on the first visit, you can't help but feel edgy, or at least on display.

He'd giggled nervously, and I'd put on my Best Professional Demeanor, nodding curtly. ("Don't let him think it matters.") I've forgotten what he was in for that first time—foot fungus? Something simple. We'd gotten through it fine.

Now he was back with blood in his semen, which was more fraught territory. He was trying, though, and I was trying. It was less uncomfortable than the guy the week before who wouldn't meet my eyes at all, but kept laughing nervously and staring at the corners of the room. "My wife made me come in," he'd said. He listed half a dozen concerns without seeming very interested in any of them, and had a hand on the doorknob before he finally blurted out his reason for being there: "My wife thinks you should give me some of that Viagra stuff."

I said, "Do you think that's something you would like to try?"

He said, "My wife would sure appreciate it if you thought so."

The gentleman with blood in his semen was trying not to blush and forcing himself to meet my eyes, even though his eyebrows were twitching wildly and I could see the thought written in bold letters across his forehead: *I'm telling the girl doc what's going on with my genitals!* He was a decent guy, and he was suppressing the thought as fast as it popped up, probably reminding himself that I had done okay with the foot fungus, or whatever it was.

He said, "I've been having a little pain when I urinate."

I put on my best serious/analytical expression and said, "How long has it been going on?"

"Three weeks, on and off."

"Tell me about your other symptoms."

"Well, a couple of weeks ago there was a drop of blood in my shorts."

I nodded, and he blurted out, "Well, and over the weekend, my wife and I were traveling and—" He looked suddenly confused. "No, that's not important." He paused to regroup. "I had the opportunity to identify that there was blood in my semen."

He was so dismayed, between the problem itself and the embarrassment of talking about it, and I was so anxious to say and do the right thing, that the moment was almost comical. Two adults, generally comfortable and mature, caught in a dizzying display of self-consciousness.

Part of my mind flashed back to when I was a third-year medical student, all of twenty-two years old, and had to do my very first testicular exam as part of a routine physical on a fourteen-year-old boy— I thought he was going to perish of embarrassment on the spot, and I was little better. Another part of me was desperately sifting through my arsenal of words, trying to find the gracious thing to say or do at this moment, to diffuse the tension while acknowledging his anxiety. A final fragment of my mind wanted to step back and note the theatrical situation, both of us trying so hard—as if we were both students, earnestly acting out a pretend clinical scenario. I wanted to step out of character and say, "Wow, this is awkward, isn't it?"

Instead I was putting on my most serious frown—to acknowledge the gravity of the experience for him, to show that I understood how frightening it was to discover blood unexpectedly in one's bodily fluids. Also to reassure him that I was not going to giggle; I suspected this was his deepest darkest fear in this moment—to tell the girl doctor about the blood and have her laugh. Quickly, though, I discarded this expression in favor of a less dark, more analytical sort of frown; I didn't want him to think that I thought that he had cancer, which, of course, was his even deeper darker fear. I worked through different degrees of frown, now strenuously keeping the edges of my lips from rising, since the whole frown conundrum was itself making me want to laugh.

"Have you had any fevers?" I asked blandly.

"No," he said, sounding relieved—whether at giving a negative reply, or just at having a yes/no question to work with, I didn't know.

"Any penile discharge?"

"No."

"Any new sexual partners?"

"No."

I knew he was married, so I added, "I'm sorry, I have to ask . . ."

"No no, it's fine, I understand."

"Any back pain or change in your bowels?"

"No."

"Okay, let's have a look at you."

I listened carefully to his heart and lungs, not because they were especially relevant, but because it was easier to move from a more general to a more focused exam, rather than go right for the genitals, as it were. I talked him through what I was checking for, using the male-genital-exam speech I've become practiced at since that first dreadful day with the fourteen-year-old. "Now I'm going to check your testicles. The surface of the testicle should feel like a boiled egg; you should check them yourself periodically, and look for any lumps. . . ."

The exam itself was not particularly awkward, after all that. Afterward I left him alone to get dressed while I flopped down on the chair in my office, oddly exhausted and wiping sweat off my brow.

I went back to the exam room and found him looking much more comfortable in his shirt and trousers. I waved him from the exam table to the chair, where he looked more comfortable still.

I explained that he probably had prostatitis. "I thought maybe that was it," he admitted, sounding relieved. "I found it on the Web—"

There were a few other things we'd rule out, I explained, but then we'd try some antibiotics and he should get better.

He nodded brightly. I handed him a lab slip and a prescription, and asked if he had any other questions.

"No, I think you've answered everything."

He offered me a hand to shake and only then did I allow myself to smile. "It's good to see you," I said.

"It's good to see you, too."

A month later he was back on my schedule, with no complaint written down this time. Oh, no, I thought. The blood isn't better, and now I've lost all credibility.

Suppressing a cringe, I walked in.

"I fell skiing and twisted my ankle," he announced, with a sheepish smile.

I smiled back. "Let's have a look."

FAMILY HISTORY

6. LIVING LONG ENOUGH

Though I was caught up at first in the details of starting practice, it wasn't long before the greater challenges of medicine rose to the forefront of my mind. Both the fascination and the frustration of doctoring lie in its unpredictability. Behind every exam room door is a medical problem to be solved and a person in need of help. The problem may be trivial, catastrophic, or anything in between. The person may be a joy and inspiration or a challenge; sometimes they'll be all in quick succession. The infinite variability of both patient and disease is what keeps doctors coming to work every day, and what keeps us awake at night.

The first time I saw Liz Williams, one of my routine questions was about her calcium intake. She fixed me with a glare from behind her thick fifties-style blue glasses. "People in my family don't live long enough to get osteoporosis," she declared.

She was a little over forty, tall, thin but heavy-boned, with a broad Germanic face that was striking rather than pretty. She had the awkwardness of tall women who have not quite achieved comfort with their height (I can say this, being one myself), a little slouched, her shoulders pulled in slightly. She wore a beautiful draping blue wool coat and the blue glasses, at once stylish and odd. She had come in for vague abdominal pain—sometimes high in her belly, sometimes low, sometimes in front and sometimes more to the back. She was transferring care from another doctor because she felt like he had lost interest in her problems. She'd had a huge workup—lots of labs, CT scans, a colonoscopy to look at her colon, and an endoscopy to look at her stomach and upper intestines, everything short of cutting open her belly and looking inside. None of the tests showed anything abnormal.

My heart sank as she reported this. I'd only been in practice a few months, but already I'd heard more stories like this than I could count: vague symptoms, in no particular pattern, getting neither better nor worse, and lots of negative tests. I doubted I would find a more satisfactory answer for her. Sometimes you do all the tests and there's nothing to find, and all you can do is reassure the patient that it isn't anything terrible, treat the pain as best you can, and wait either for it to get better or for her to learn to live with it. Of course, I would go carefully through her records. We would watch for anything that might have been missed or unexplored, reevaluate anything that was changing. I knew and respected her prior doctor, though, and I doubted there would be any stones that hadn't already been turned.

I expected we would repeat some of the tests, find nothing new, try more tests. She would be in and out of my office for months, certain we were missing something desperately wrong. I would end up saying, "We've looked at everything there is to look at. I believe your pain is real but I can reassure you it isn't something dangerous, and beyond that there isn't any more we can do." Perhaps we would end up in arguments about pain medicines: she, wanting anything that might make her feel a little better; I, afraid of adding addiction and side effects to the problems she already had. Then she would leave me, like she left her last doctor, saying that I didn't listen or I didn't take her seriously, and I would feel terrible, and just a little bit relieved.

My future with Liz flashed before me in an instant, more an

instinct than an articulated thought. I pushed it aside; we would try, we would hope to find an answer. But I couldn't quite suppress the sour feeling in my stomach, the fear that this story would end badly.

I asked her about depression. Some people with vague abdominal pain are depressed; we rarely know which causes which, but sometimes the pain will get better if the depression is treated.

"Of course, I'm depressed," she said, irritably. She'd always been somewhat depressed, and had gotten more so since her divorce a few years earlier. One of her sisters had recently died in a car accident. She'd moved here from California to get away from her family and her ex-husband.

She told me she was thinking about moving back again. "Something like this—like having this pain—makes you really think about who your true friends are. Who will really be there when you need them, who will stick it out with you, versus who is just there because it's convenient, or because they get something out of you. The minute you have something difficult going on or you need them, they start to see you as a liability and disappear." She snorted. "I feel like I'm continually auditioning: 'Am I fun enough to be your friend? Here, let me be more *likable*.'"

As she spoke I found myself wondering where I fit, as a doctor and a person. If she were my friend instead of my patient, would I be there for her? As her physician, with a problem that I feared I wouldn't find a cause or cure for—would I be there for her in the way that she needed, or wouldn't I? What did it say about me either way?

"So many relationships in life are so superficial," she continued. "You try to get beyond that, to go to a deeper level, and people get uncomfortable. I was trying to talk to my sister—even with people you've known your whole life you can get caught into this *how's the weather, what did you do today* stuff, and never really talk. But I'll say something like, 'I feel so alone,' and she'll say, 'Well, we're all really alone in a way, aren't we, Liz,' and then go on to something else. Whatever. It's not her thing I guess. But really—"

She made a face.

I reviewed her tests, which had been very thorough. I repeated her labs to make sure nothing had changed. Everything was normal. We decided to recheck an ultrasound—maybe they'd missed something in the earlier scans? I was reaching for anything, glad just to have something to do. It showed a little gallbladder sludge, though no signs of obstruction or infection. Her pancreatic duct looked a little big, but the radiologist commented that CT scans show the duct more accurately, and she'd had a normal one just before she transferred care to me.

"Sludge," Liz said during our follow-up visit. "Isn't that a ridiculous word? I thought the technician was kidding when he said: 'We see some sludge.' It sounds like a garbage-man word, not a doctor word."

I remember laughing at the term, too, when I first heard it, but, like so many lay terms we use differently in medical parlance, it's ceased to seem comic or even odd to me.

I sent her to a surgeon, who scheduled her to have the gallbladder removed. She was thrilled. "I'm just so glad we've found something. That we're going to get it out and make the pain go away."

My own excitement at having a potential culprit was more tempered. "Remember, there's a chance that this may not be it, that we'll take the gallbladder out and you'll still have the pain—"

"I know," she said. "But still. We're doing something."

It was a Wednesday night, the week before her scheduled surgery. A colleague with season tickets to the Seattle Sonics had given me his expensive seats. It had been a hard week—I'd been covering several hospital patients for a vacationing colleague, adding an exhausting extra hour to each end of my day. My colleague had just returned and I was relieved at the thought of not having anyone in the hospital, no extra visits to make before and after clinic, and fewer late-night calls. Just after halftime in the game my pager went off, flashing a hospital number, the floor of two patients I had been covering.

I found a quietish back hallway in the stadium and dialed the number. I was almost looking forward to saying, "I'd love to help you but Dr. Alberts is back in town, and this is his patient, so why don't you give him a call?"

But the voice was one of my clinic's gastroenterologists. "Emily, do you have a couple minutes? It's about a patient of yours, Liz Williams."

It took me a moment to reorient my thoughts.

"Liz Williams who's going to have her gallbladder out next Monday?"

"Liz Williams who had her gallbladder out yesterday," he said. "Her pain got suddenly worse, so they moved it up. Nobody called you?"

"No."

"I figured they hadn't, or you would have come. Anyway, they got in there and her gallbladder was all matted up and necrotic. They got it out, but they thought just from the look of it that things were pretty bad. The pathology report just came back, and it's adenocarcinoma. Not clear if the cancer started in her gallbladder or pancreas. Not good either way."

I flashed back to a day when I was a chief resident, and one of our most thorough and insightful junior residents presented a case at our morning conference. "This one isn't very interesting," he said, "but it's a useful thought experiment." He went on to describe a young woman with vomiting and extreme weight loss. The group ran through the list of all the things this could be, the tests that needed to be done.

"She's pretty depressed, and I think it's anorexia," the resident said at the end. "But it's useful to think about all the things it *could* have been. They're looking down with a scope at her esophagus tomorrow, just in case." He shrugged. "Have to do it, but not much chance we'll find anything."

The next day he was in my office almost in tears, after the endoscopy showed a huge tumor eating away the young woman's esophagus.

"I didn't believe it," he said. "I thought it was just anorexia. I didn't believe it was something else."

"You didn't have to," I told him. "You did what you were supposed to do. You got the endoscopy, to make sure, and you found it. That's what workups are for. It's not your job to make the right guess; it's your job to do the right thing. You did."

He shook his head. "I didn't believe it," he said, choking on the words.

"I know," I said. "But that's okay."

Did I still believe that now?

"Hey," I said, at her bedside an hour later. I'd left the game, gone home to change before I came to the hospital. I walked into her room having no idea where she might be emotionally, if she'd be angry or in denial or in despair. Not knowing what I could do to help, I waited to see what she would say.

She put on her blue glasses and scrunched up her nose. "It's been quite a week," she said.

I smiled at her dryness, pulled up a chair, and sat down. "So I hear. Do you want to talk about it?"

"I don't know," she said. "It's all a jumble."

I nodded and waited for more.

"When I first moved here, I was in this therapy group. There was a woman there who had moved to Seattle a year or two earlier, and soon after she came she was diagnosed with breast cancer. She was doing fine; she had surgery and she was over it, pretty much. And she said: 'Seattle is a great place to get cancer.'"

Liz made another of her wonderful scrunched-face expressions. "I mean—I don't think she meant anything all that strange by it. And it's probably true. But still, it seemed like such an odd thing to say."

She thought for a moment.

"I think she meant, there are all these programs and everything, and the Hutchinson Cancer Center, and so on."

I nodded.

"Still, it seemed like such a strange thing to say, in a conversation, you know. . . . 'Seattle is a great place to get cancer.' And now—well, we'll see, I guess."

There was a long pause, after which we chatted about small things. I'd read the book on her bedside table; she mentioned that the author was giving a reading soon. We got into a conversation about readings, fiction and poetry, things we'd seen and missed.

"You know who was just wonderful, was Donald Hall. I saw him last year, a beautiful reading, every word just straight from the heart. He had a very touching poem about the nurses here at this hospital. His wife was treated here. She was a poet, too—Jane Kenyon. She had some kind of cancer."

"Leukemia," I said absently, surprised. I love her poetry, especially her searing, insightful poems about depression. I hadn't known that she was treated here.

"Yes. Yes, that's it—"

She looked at me with strange intensity, as if I had just said the first intelligible thing in our whole relationship. Perhaps I had finally proved myself to be of some value. She surveyed me with new interest.

"She wrote beautiful poems," I said.

"Yes. He read a bunch of them. More of hers than his own, actually."

I felt a terrible stab of loss. I had missed Jane Kenyon's husband reading her words.

"It's a good town for poetry. Lots of readings, lots of interest. Not every city has an all-poetry bookstore, for instance. Seattle even has a poetry press."

"A good town for poetry, and cancer?" I asked.

I regretted the words the moment they were out of my mouth, but she giggled. "Even the two together. A good town for poetry and cancer. Poetry-N-Cancer."

While we talked, she was drinking contrast for a CT scan. Her surgeon called me the next morning with the results. There were four spots in her liver that hadn't been there on her scan two months ago. Metastases.

I came back that afternoon, and found her gastroenterologist and surgeon standing, one in a white coat and the other in scrubs, at the foot of her bed. I dropped to a crouch at Liz's bedside and took her hand. She squeezed my fingers and didn't let go, although she was still talking to the surgeon. I remained in my crouch.

"I'm not talking about miracles," she was saying. "I haven't ruled that out, as it happens, but it's not what I want to talk about right now.

"I'm just trying to understand the words you're using, to get a grasp on the terminology. When you just said that the cancer is not 'resectable for cure,' that 'cure is not an option,' but you talk about 'treating' with radiation or chemotherapy—"

The surgeon cleared his throat. "The only way to get rid of the cancer completely would be to cut it out, and get clean margins. To cut it out and get it all, you understand. These spots in your liver. . . . Assuming they are what we think they are, they're in too many places. Both lobes of the liver. That means we can't cut them out."

She nodded. "These spots."

"Yes?"

"You keep saying they look like metastases. But you can't tell until you—what did you say?—'look at the tissue.' "

"Yes."

"What else could they be?"

"That's what they look like. I think it's overwhelmingly likely that that's what they are."

"But. . . ."

The gastroenterologist spoke from the back of the room. "Cysts. Clusters of blood vessels. Things like that."

Liz nodded.

"But they look like metastases," the surgeon repeated.

"So in that case—"

"In that case cure is not an option, and we would be looking at palliative measures."

"So you're saying I'm going to—" She paused, waving her hand in the air abstractly, searching for a word. At last she found it: "—Die—" She said it in a tone that was at once dramatic and matter-of-fact, with another flourish of her hand; as if this were on the one hand an accepted truth, and on the other a rather histrionic way of putting things. As if the word was boring, trite. *You're saying I'm going to die, if you will—.* Almost a roll of her eyes as she tossed the word out into the room.

It was the exact opposite of the way I would have used the word, gently and gingerly, fearing it contained too much. "Die. . . ." Such a tiny syllable, to hold so much.

"These other things, radiation, chemotherapy, would be—"

"Chemotherapy and radiation would be ways to cut down on the bulk of the tumor, to treat the pain potentially, to make it grow more slowly."

"So the goal is . . . ?"

Neither the surgeon nor the gastroenterologist said anything.

"To buy you time," I said.

There was an interminable pause. Then she nodded, and I thought I saw her shrug. "So, when can I go home?"

"We can figure out the next step as an outpatient," the surgeon said. "There's nothing keeping you here, unless you feel more comfortable—"

"I'd rather not stay," she said curtly.

"Tomorrow, then," he said. My mind drifted, trying to follow the nuances of her tone, to imagine her thoughts. While I pondered, the surgeon was reviewing the list of medications she would take home. Pain pills, stomach-acid blockers, iron. "Your blood counts have dropped a little, and you need to build them up again."

She frowned. "Won't iron interfere with my calcium? Dr. Transue put me on calcium for my bones, and I thought that didn't go with iron."

She was looking at the surgeon, and I was glad she didn't see my involuntary flinch. He glanced toward me: "Medication interactions are your department." I had schooled my expression by the time I met her eyes.

"Let's stop the calcium for a while."

She nodded distractedly—point settled, on to the next thing—and I had a flash of relief that her quick mind was too distracted to see beneath my words. Her words at our first meeting echoed back, horrifyingly prescient. "People in my family don't live long enough to get osteoporosis."

The surgeon and the gastroenterologist left, and I stayed with her, still kneeling and holding her hand.

"Liz—I'm sorry."

I wasn't sure whether I was apologizing or expressing sorrow, or why: for not having found out earlier what was wrong, for not being able to cure her, for not having believed there was something terrible causing her pain? Or a simpler, more human sorrow: that this was happening, that she was going to die.

"I'm looking forward just to being home."

"Yes."

"Actually it will be the first time I've had in months with the pain—what's the word my nurse used earlier? It wasn't 'controlled,' it was—'managed.'"

I didn't have an answer to the rebuke implicit in her words.

She sat in silence for a while, leaving me with my thoughts and my guilt. I knew intellectually that I had done everything I was supposed to do, that even if we'd caught the cancer the first day she came to me we wouldn't have been able to cure her. Some people will die from cancer as surely as others will get hit by buses, and we will be as unable to prevent it. It didn't make me feel better. I remembered the crushing guilt of the resident who thought his patient had anorexia, and my inability to comfort him when it turned out she, too, had cancer.

Liz's voice broke in on my thoughts. "How strange, to have this happening to me. I mean—people suffer. We all know that. But you never understand it, really. I mean, why should you care, if it's not you? Really. I never really did—"

I knew she meant on a much deeper level than concern, or sympathy. She was talking more to herself than me, but I wanted to break in and say: I care. You care about others, and I care about you.

I also knew, though, that in a way she was right, that I didn't and couldn't understand. A terrible ache of loneliness radiated from her, the deep, unanswerable loneliness of the human condition.

All I could do was hold her hand, and say, again, "I'm sorry."

7. LOSS

The topic of emotional boundaries in medicine is always complicated. Doctors deal with people in some of the most emotional moments in their lives; the endless challenge is how to be present and involved in our patients' crises without being too bruised by their traumas to function and give objective advice. Meantime we, of course, have our own lives with their inherent complications. Paradoxically, bringing one's human self to the practice of medicine is essential to being a good physician, yet professionalism and good sense demand that this be kept within strict limits. Each patient deserves the best of care whether their doctor is having a good day or a bad one, and whether she finds the topic at hand easy or difficult.

Before I entered medicine, I believed that a doctor's personal and professional lives could be cleanly separate. I envisioned that I would feel deeply for my patients, care about them and their families; yet I would leave it all at the office when I went home. Likewise, the ups and downs of my outside life would be left neatly at the clinic door, to be picked up again at the end of the day. Needless to say, reality is not so simple. Emotion and life experience don't turn off with walking through a door, or donning and shedding a white coat. Grief and loss, in particular, resonate strongly across these boundaries. I grieved for Liz Williams; my sorrow at the knowledge that she was going to die stayed with me in and outside of work. Likewise, the struggles of my personal life colored my interactions with my patients. Properly channeled, painful experiences can become a powerful source of empathy, but finding this path isn't easy. The stronger the emotion, the harder the journey.

He brought her in to meet me. They were a sweet elderly couple, the woman small and frail with her hair tied back in a handkerchief, the man neatly dressed and powerfully built, both in their seventies. It was clear at a glance that he was the caregiver and she the cared-for. He helped guide her up onto the exam table, held her hand for reassurance. When I asked a question, even something as simple as why she had come in, she looked to him, with charming confidence, for guidance.

"You're here for a physical," I noted.

She nodded toward him. "Whatever he said."

"How have you been feeling?" I asked.

She turned to him for help.

"Tell her how you've been feeling," he said encouragingly.

"Fine," she said at last. "I feel fine."

I examined her. Physically, she was healthy, but she couldn't do the simplest mental tasks. She knew her name, and not much more. Afterward I talked to him alone. "She's . . ." He tapped his head, and sighed. "She's not right in the head. Well, you can see."

"How are you two managing, at home?" He'd told me they lived independently; I was amazed, guessing at her needs.

"It's hard. Well—it's really hard. She needs so much, you know. Sometimes she's fine, sometimes she's almost all there. We can have a conversation, she can get herself dressed. Other times—there's just nothing. She doesn't wander off, thank God. I can leave her for a few minutes to run to the grocery store, say, and she won't leave the house. So that's one big thing I don't have to worry about. I should be grateful. But still. It's hard."

"It's one of the hardest situations there is," I said. "Taking care of someone who's not all there, or who's in and out. Never knowing what it will be on a given day."

He nodded. "My kids and friends say I should put her someplace. But she's there enough to know she doesn't want to go."

"You're a good man to do it," I said. "You should know, though, it's probably not going to work forever." I tried to soften the hard words with a smile. "I know she wants it to, and you want it to. But she's pretty sick, and a time will come when she'll probably need professional care. It won't be safe for either of you to keep her at home."

"I know," he said. "But it's not so easy."

"It may be the hardest thing there is," I said.

"You just can't imagine."

I didn't tell him that, in fact, I could.

Medical stories have a certain structure, imbued by the structure of the doctor-patient interaction. Someone comes in with a question, a problem, a "complaint." With more or less drawing out, the patient tells a story. Information is gathered, a theory is developed, a plan is made. At each stage or visit, the doctor documents a summation in the medical record.

Family stories are different. Each piece grows out of something that has come before, every story folds in on itself and out against the future. When I was a child, my father had a magical book called *Kaleidocycles*. It was made up of prints of M. C. Escher designs, which could be cut out, then carefully folded and pasted into three-dimensional forms, mobile twisted boxes that turned in on themselves. As you rolled them, one pattern shifted into the next, wrapping finally back around to the original. Family stories are kaleidocycles, only less neat.

In its simplest form, my father's story was this. For several years in his late thirties he had headaches, progressively more frequent and severe. One day he suddenly and briefly lost his vision. He went to the ER, where a CT scan showed a tumor in his brainstem. He was taken to surgery almost immediately. The tumor, which turned out to be a cancer, was successfully removed. He was given radiation afterwards, to kill any remaining cancer cells.

It was 1981, and I was ten years old. My memories of that time are fragmented, yet painfully vivid and sometimes strangely sweet. I remember my mother's arms wrapped protectively around my brother and me, telling us the news about the man she had divorced some years before: "Your father has a cancer in his brain." Then, I remember the day of the surgery, sitting in my sixth-grade classroom, unable to concentrate on school, staring at the trees outside the window. The hospital lawn where we picnicked after the operation, eating impossibly red sweet cherries, my father alive—we had been told he might die during the procedure—bandaged but cheerful, himself. My parents, who were barely on speaking terms, sitting together and chatting affectionately in the vivid sunshine, this friendliness seeming to my young mind the biggest miracle of all.

"Is he a vegetable?" my schoolmates asked in hushed voices. The phrase still makes me cringe, though I can now find comedy in it as well, the suggestion of a brain-damaged parent as an eggplant, a rutabaga. "No," I explained. "He's not a vegetable. Not even a little bit. He's fine."

It would be a decade before it was clear that he wasn't fine. The onset of dementia was, as it so often is, subtle and befuddling. Was he slower than he had been? Did it take a maddening amount of time for him to tie his shoes or carry dishes to the table, or was that just my adolescent peevishness? The one overt complication of the surgery had been to leave him deaf in one ear, and over time the hearing in his other ear ebbed a little. Expensive hearing aids were little help. When he receded from a conversation into his own world, or seemed not to understand what was happening around him, was it just a consequence of the deafness? The damaged ear affected his balance; was he so slow because he was afraid to fall, and had slowness then just deepened into habit? Of course, with his history, the doctors did tests. The labs, the CTs and the MRIs were negative; if there was something wrong, it wasn't cancer.

I was a teenager. My parents had separated when I was six and divorced when I was eight. My brother and I lived with my mother, spending alternate weekends with my father for some years, and vacations with him and my grandparents. I adored my father, but we weren't close in a day-to-day way. He lived in another city; neither of us was good about writing letters or calling often. He brought me lovely, thoughtful presents from places that he traveled. He would hear a nice piece on the piano and send me the music. He liked to teach me things. I remember sitting at his kitchen table when I was eight or nine while he taught me math games, showing me how to figure out a missing number in an ever more complicated series of puzzles. We called the mystery number "x," and only years later would I realize that the puzzles were equations and the topic algebra.

It was my mother, though, who raised me. My father's presence in my life, though bright, was small, even in the years before the cancer and the apparently healthy years soon afterward. The weekend visits tapered off as my brother and I got older and didn't like to leave our friends. During the time when it was becoming clear that he wasn't well, I was busy with adolescent things, growing up, not paying much attention to my father's health.

Nerve cells are delicate. We—I use the word as a member of the medical profession, always an uneasy role in connection to my father—know a great deal now that we didn't know in 1981, or even 1991. We understand now that some tissues can survive radiation better than others, that brain tissue in particular tends to develop delicate internal webs of scar over time after heavy radiation exposure. After too much irradiation, particularly the doses used long ago before the amount and direction were as finely tuned as they are now, the brain could subtly—and later, sometimes, catastrophically—lose function. "Encephalopathy," it's called, or "encephalomalacia." Latin for "wrongness in the head." Over the years after his treatment, my father's brain slowly turned to scar.

The shape of a tragedy can vary from the instantaneous—a healthy teenager killed in a car accident, a baby's death by SIDS—to the terribly prolonged, the slow but inexorable growth of certain cancers, the brain-cell-by-brain-cell decline of dementia. The most abrupt and the most prolonged losses are terrible in distinct ways. Though many people want to go quickly when the time comes, it helps to have time to prepare, both for the person dying and for their loved ones. An unexpected loss can leave many things undone and unsaid. Death is a shock in any form, but sudden ones rattle the worlds of the survivors more, remind us of our own mortality: *I could be there a moment hence . . .*

Slow decline has its own cruelties. Many people with cancer or heart failure or lung disease suffer pain and breathlessness. The medical profession can do a great deal to soothe pain and to ease breathing, but not everything. Dementia twists its knife differently, not the vital functions of the body but those of the mind ravaged by illness. Few things in the world are harder than watching someone you love fade bit by bit, the body remaining but the person inside little by little ceasing to exist.

In the landscape of my father's illness, the many dark years of descent, there are certain moments that stand out in my memory. I visited him and my grandparents in Maine one summer when I was in college. He mentioned, rather casually, that he was trying to figure out what the things were that flew in the trees but didn't have wings. He didn't think they made any noise, although he pointed out reasonably that he saw them primarily at night when his hearing aids weren't in, so he realized that they might make sounds he couldn't hear. I was a biology major, so he thought I might have some ideas about them.

I tried to ask more questions. What did they look like? How big were they? What did he mean by flying without wings? Did they float? Were their wings so fast they couldn't be seen, like a bee's or a hummingbird's?

He was clear on the negatives and murky on the positives. They weren't birds, or insects. They flew, they didn't float. No wings at all. They were somewhat square in shape. At last he confessed he had concluded they might be UFOs.

I laughed. I thought it was a joke; my father disbelieved equally in God and the paranormal. I continued to puzzle over what his creatures might be—surely there was a reasonable explanation—fighting the realization that in fact they were hallucinations. If I acknowledged that, I would have to acknowledge the deeper truth, that something was terribly wrong. Up to that time he had just been slow—might a man not be forgiven for being slow, after everything he'd been through? In retrospect there had been other things that clearly weren't right, but the UFOs, for me, were the breakthrough, the shard that finally began to pierce my thick layers of denial.

Another vivid moment was also in Maine, a few years later. My grandparents had bought land there when my father was young, and we spent a part of the summer there every year of my childhood. It was on the far northern coast, close to the Canadian border, and the ocean was very cold. Few people swam in it, except for my grandmother, who swam almost every day; whenever I was there, I went with her. From the time I was very small I had a reputation as a cold-water fish; I could swim as far out as our sailboat mooring and back again, staying in the water until I was blue and numb, teeth chattering. There is still a scar across my forehead, acquired when I was five years old. I had swum until I was half frozen, and was walking up the rocky beach so tightly wrapped in my towel that I couldn't put my hands out to brace myself when I tripped. I gashed my forehead on a jagged stone, and bled profusely in my father's lap on the long drive to the nearest emergency room, where they sewed me up with twenty-three tiny stitches. This incident did not cure my swimming habit.

Twenty years later I walked on the same beach with my ailing father, keeping an arm under his elbow to steady him; the rocks were sharp as ever and his balance was not so good. He walked in short, unsteady steps on the uneven ground. We made our way down to the water, stepping carefully across the kelp and algae since the tide was low, and dipped our toes into the ocean.

"It's cold," he said. His words had become like his steps, slower and fewer.

"Yes. Cold as ever," I answered.

He smiled at me, with tenderness but also an odd uncertainty. "Have you ever swum in it?" he asked.

I could point to any number of other moments that whispered the same message. On a snowy night the winter before, he fussed that I might try to go outside without my shoes on—I was in my twenties by then, a medical student. The next day he frowned when I got out my car keys, and asked if I had ever driven in the snow, as though my young adulthood in the snowy regions of Ohio and New England had never happened. Unready to hear, I laughed it off—a father's protectiveness. Parents always think of their children as, well, children, don't they? But mine really didn't know whether I knew to put on my shoes. Now, little by little, he was forgetting me. In the murky folds and shadows of his slowly disintegrating brain, the concept of me—who I was, who I had been, the little girl paddling beside her grandmother in the salt water, the screaming child bleeding into his lap, the serious student, the pianist, the avid reader, everything that made up the essential entity of myself, as well as all the other things and people he knew—was being lost.

By the time I started my medical practice, he had forgotten my name. Like so many things in dementia, it came and went for a while, until finally it was gone completely. There were times when he would recognize me as someone familiar, sometimes clearly precious, other times a complete unknown. Once, he seemed not to recognize me at all, then leaned across to someone we walked past and confided:

"She's a *very* close relative."

Dementia has its comic moments, albeit a very dark form of comedy. I could smile at that, even as my eyes filled with tears. "*Daughter*," I said. "I'm your daughter."

I'd had many years, by that time, of little losses and little grievings. This is the peculiar quality of dementia, that you lose someone bit by bit instead of all at once, and live your grief in a series of small, unrelenting losses. All of us who loved him had gone through more stages of grief than Elisabeth Kübler-Ross could list or we could name. I remember the strange, empty moment when I let go of anger, my pointless anger at the world for his illness and my irrational, guilty anger at him for being sick, but also all the normal angers that children have at parents. It was a cold, sunny day in the courtyard of the nursing home where he lived then, with light streaming down on the flower boxes full of geraniums. The realization came over me that I would never have a chance to take him to task for the small betrayals of fatherhood—not being there during times I thought I needed him; letting me and my brother get painfully caught in the middle of his bitter divorce from my mother; not answering the desperate advice-seeking letter I sent him in the midst of some romantic crisis in college. Oddly, the letting-go of anger itself was a loss; I longed for that normal, healthy anger, the silly righteous irritation at small wrongs, real or perceived. It was strangely terrible to face how pointless all those normal feelings were, how little they connected to the empty husk of a man in front of me. I forgave, if there was anything to forgive; yet I lost more in that moment than in the moment he forgot my name.

I think the hardest of all, though, was on the beach with the cold lapping waves. "Have you ever swum in it?" *You don't know me. You are my father and you don't know me.*

I said none of this to the husband of my demented patient. I didn't say I knew the way he felt, since of course I couldn't. I barely knew the way I felt with my father in any given moment; how could I imagine how it was for someone else?

"It's hard," was all I said. "I know it's very, very hard."

8. GODIVA DIABETIC

After about six months in practice, as my anxiety over whether I knew how to do my job faded, I discovered a different kind of challenge: the overwhelming effort of being present with patient after patient, day after day, remaining attentive to their needs and sensitive to their points of view. It struck me that this shift from the "acute" to the "chronic" work of doctoring paralleled the experience of patients in dealing with acute versus chronic illness. For someone with a life-threatening infection, the moment of crisis may be terrible, but everything then goes back to normal. For someone with diabetes or arthritis, death is not an immediate danger; but the prospect of a life spent accommodating and fighting the disease—weaving it into the way one eats, drinks, moves—can be more difficult than any brief catastrophe.

It was the final day of a hard week. I'd been on call and very busy the weekend before, so I'd worked twelve consecutive long days without ever feeling I could catch my breath. I was thrilled that I had finally made it to Friday afternoon, and I wanted nothing more than to turn off my pager and get into my car and drive home. I was fantasizing about a cold beer, and Chinese food, and bed.

My last patient of the afternoon was labeled, on the "complaint" line of the schedule, "New patient/Diabetes/Depression/Pain all over."

In addition to seeing her, I had to deal with a pile of phone messages on my desk before I could leave. "Personal, needs call tonight," from a patient I talked to about some new perceived crisis three times a week. There was another message from someone I spent half an hour talking to on Tuesday about how glad he was to finally be off drugs after three weeks of inpatient rehab treatment. Now the message said that he was forced to do a random drug test on Wednesday and he actually had used cocaine, "just a little," on Saturday—before the appointment where he told me he was clean—and would they be able to detect that? "Please call back ASAP."

Leaving all these things on my desk, I went in to see New patient/Diabetes/Depression/Pain all over.

She was a small woman, plump and pretty, with her thin black hair a little teased. She smelled like powder, and looked like one of the women my grandmother plays bridge with.

"It looks like we have a lot to talk about today," I said, summoning all my energies. I reminded myself that the last patient of the week deserved no less attention than the first, and tried to be the doctor I'd want my grandmother's friend to have. "Why don't you start by telling me a little about yourself?"

Thread by thread her story spooled. She'd been divorced years before—this was when her depression began, as well as her overeating. Her new boyfriend, whom she adored, didn't understand why she still struggled with being sad, and she was afraid to admit to him that in fact she was sick, too. He didn't know she was diabetic, although she'd been diagnosed more than ten years before. She wasn't taking any medication, didn't follow her blood sugars. Her cholesterol was extremely high; her mother's had been, too, and she'd died young of heart disease. The more she thought about her health, the sadder she was, and the sadder she was the more she ate. On top of that, lately everything had started to hurt. She said she hated doctors (I smiled, thinking of my grandmother), but she had come to me because she just didn't know how to get through the day anymore.

Hot tears flowed out of her cool green eyes and down her powdered cheeks.

"It's very hard," I said, when her story finally came to a close. "Trying to deal with all these things must be very hard."

She cut me short. "I know I have to deal with all of it. I've been told before, you don't have to tell me again. If I don't I'm going to have to go on dialysis and get my feet cut off and die."

I was a little shocked by this harsh assessment. "Well—it's true that all of those things can be long-term consequences of diabetes, and that's why we have to help you get it under control. But that's a pretty overwhelming way to think about it. We both know why it's important; let's just tackle it one little piece at a time."

She looked up at me, a little brighter.

"This is going to be a day-by-day thing. We're going to have to make changes in your life in a way that you can accept, can live with."

"It's just so hard to try to accept that I'm never going to get to eat another chocolate. . . ." Her voice caught and broke on the word "chocolate."

I frowned. I'm not a big fan of the term "never," though it has its uses. I had a patient who had his esophagus taken out for cancer, and he was truly never going to eat another chocolate, or anything else. When an alcoholic chooses never to have another drink, more power to them. But most things in medicine, as in the rest of life, aren't that black and white—including a diabetic's diet.

"I don't think you need to feel like you're never going to eat another chocolate," I suggested. "Diabetes—" I paused to organize my thoughts. "Diabetes is a terrible disease, it can cause terrible problems. Over the long run we need to keep it as well controlled as we can, as much of the time as we can. I won't lie to you, that's very difficult. Still. . . . It's about balances and averages, not about absolute rules. You certainly shouldn't eat sugar very much or very often. But 'never' is a strong word."

"What am I supposed to do, then?"

"You have to find the balance that works for you, to keep you healthy but happy, too. Don't ever eat something that's bad for you unless you really, truly want to. When you are going to have a chocolate, make it a darn good chocolate, and just have one. Don't do it too often. That's different from thinking you never can."

She looked at me like I just lifted a death sentence, rather than just suggesting the use of common sense. "Really?"

"Really."

"How did you put that? 'Don't ever eat something that's bad for you that you don't really want.' I'm going to remember that."

"I didn't mean it to be anything profound."

She countered, "I read this book. . . . It was by a doctor who was diabetic. It said: You have eaten your last piece of cake. Your last chocolate, your last piece of candy. It said: You can have eggs and sausages for breakfast, but you will never again have an orange."

I don't know whether the book actually said that; it doesn't really matter. What mattered was what she heard, and the fact that it overwhelmed her to a point where she couldn't face the problem at all.

"Let's take a different kind of approach," I suggested.

She needed to be on something for her high blood pressure: ironically, controlling blood pressure, which she hadn't given a thought to, is as important to reducing diabetic complications as controlling blood sugar, which was making her so unhappy. She needed medication for her high cholesterol. But we decided to start instead with treatment for her depression, since fixing that would make everything else easier to tackle. There was a stack of other things she needed: an eye exam for diabetic eye damage, urine tests for her kidneys, half a dozen blood tests, a mammogram, a screening colonoscopy. None of these was urgent, so we would put them off until another time. In the bigger picture, she would need to decide how to tell her boyfriend about her health issues. He adored her and I felt sure that he would be supportive, whereas her current efforts to hide her health from him were just adding to her stress.

I made her a list of the things we would be doing between now and her next visit, to make sure she understood and remembered them. I tried to keep the list simple and short; there were lots of pieces to deal with, but we would address them one at a time. As we got to my last item, though, she sniffled. I looked up and realized she was crying.

"I'm so sorry," I said. "I didn't mean to overwhelm you. I know it's a lot of things to be thinking about at once."

"No, no, it's not that."

She blew her nose.

"It's just . . . it's just that it's nice to know that someone is going to help me deal with all this." She laughed wearily. "You probably think I've been sent here as a test. A plant, last thing on a Friday afternoon—. You're probably thinking, where did this crazy person come from, and why is she doing this to me? . . ."

I smiled, because although I had been thinking something rather along those lines before I walked into the room, I'd actually enjoyed the visit. "Actually—" I wasn't sure how to say this without seeming callous. "Actually this is why I went into this field. I like doing this. This—feels good."

She smiled shyly. "It feels good to me, too."

"Good. Back in two weeks, then?"

"Yes."

As she stood at the front desk making her follow-up appointment, I went back into my office. It was late, and my desk was still piled high with charts and papers. Yet, returning the phone calls from the person with the every-other-day crises and the man with the positive drug test suddenly didn't seem all that bad. I got a glimpse of how one might stay happy and fulfilled in medicine, even when it seemed overwhelming. Just as the challenges of practice were analogous to the challenges of chronic illness, the solution was similar, too. Keep tackling one problem at a time, and treasure each little reward along the way. With renewed heart, I picked up the telephone.

9. LOST AND FOUND

Medicine is not only about taking care of individuals, it's about families, the dynamics of interlaced lives. Sometimes my patients' greatest health crises happened not in their own lives but in the ones around them, just as my father's health issues were a greater force in my life than my own. For others, like my Godiva Diabetic, loved ones could be either a help or a hindrance, depending on how they were brought into the picture. Observing the dynamics of families is one of the great fascinations of my work—watching couples interact, parents and children, partners and friends. I witness the spectrum from tender to sad, from supportive to destructive, and sometimes all of the above in a single pair.

One of my favorite couples, Ellie and George, appeared in my office for the first time during a blizzard, or what passes for a blizzard in Seattle. There were seven inches of snow on the ground and the city was completely shut down. It was my first winter in practice but my fifth in Seattle, and I'd never seen so much snow here. All the schools and the highways were closed. I skidded my car across two miles of deserted streets to get to the clinic, and sat in an empty office all morning as patient after patient called to announce they weren't coming. I worked through mounds of paperwork and embraced the idea that it would be a day without patients. Then, like an apparition out of the storm, in they came, two bent snowswept figures in tattered jackets, smelling of fresh snowy air with heavy overtones of beer.

They'd stumbled up through the snow the several blocks from their apartment. Once I'd got over my astonishment—my seventy-year-old new patient showed up, in this weather, for a routine checkup?—and once they'd thawed a little, we settled into the room to talk.

They were both completely drunk. Words I don't usually use drifted through my mind: "soused"; "hammered." The husband was very charming, like the aging military veteran he was, and she was charmingly crabby. She answered every question with a quick, sharp retort, but a little giggle frequently seeped through around the edges. I liked her immediately.

She was in surprisingly good health, little the worse for the wear of advanced age and self-neglect. I ran through her medical history and uncovered little. "Have you ever been pregnant?" I asked.

"No."

Her husband leaned in confidentially. "She was a virgin when I met her fifteen years ago."

"George, you didn't have to tell her that!" she said, and hit him with her cane.

I asked how much she drank and they both giggled.

"I don't know. . . . Maybe a six-pack . . ."

"Maybe before lunch!" Her husband tittered, and she hit him again.

"Ask her about her dogs," my medical assistant whispered, lifting her hand to her mouth to cover a smile, when I stepped out into the hall to get a lab slip. She had a wonderful way of getting personal tidbits from people in the minutes she spent checking them in and taking vital signs.

"Tell me about your dogs," I said when I went back in.

"Oh, we've got two," Ellie said demurely.

"Mine is named Fat Bastard," the husband announced brightly.

"And mine is Rotten."

Afterward, I rather wondered if I'd imagined them both, the happy drunken senior citizens from out of the snow. But she came back now and again with one small problem or another, invariably drunk and invariably irritable, but in an oddly endearing way. After a few visits she seemed to decide that she liked me also. The day she hugged me as she said good-bye, I felt like a queen on earth.

My coverage system was set up so that I took calls from my own patients on weeknights, but on weekends there was rotating call among eight internists. When I wasn't on call, the weekend ended on Sunday night at nine o'clock, when my pager went back on and the covering doc from the weekend called to tell me about my patients in the hospital. One Sunday night, Ellie was on the list.

"She came in on Saturday morning with pneumonia," the covering doctor said. "Drunk—can you imagine being falling-down drunk at age seventy, at nine in the morning no less? I put her on some antibiotics, she's doing a little better. She should go home in a day or two."

Yes, if we can keep her out of alcohol withdrawal, I thought with a sinking heart. Ironically, the hospital might be a more dangerous place for her than home.

By the next day, in spite of medication to try to ward off withdrawal, she was in its early stages: delirious, incontinent, and screaming. When I walked into her room on Monday morning she didn't recognize me; she howled when I came near. I wondered if it would have been possible to treat her pneumonia at home, where she could continue her usual drinking habit—not healthy, of course, but safer than stopping suddenly—instead of bringing her into the hospital. It wouldn't have been the textbook thing to do in a frail seventy-year-old, and probably I wouldn't have dared—bacteria could have spread from her lungs to her blood, and she could have died. On the other hand, she might have done fine; instead we were faced with this.

For two solid weeks she screamed. She howled at the nurses, she howled at me, she wailed with every blood draw and blood-pressure check. She howled at her husband, who crumpled against the wall and wept, my arms awkwardly around his shoulders.

I could hear her every morning as I stepped off the elevator onto the ward. My heart would sink and a wave of nausea would wash over me when I heard the familiar cries. I accepted meekly the curious and irritated glares of staff and families and physicians as I headed toward her room.

"Can't you . . . ?"

"No. I can't."

I gave her enough sedatives to knock out a polar bear, enough Haldol to silence Cassandra, and still she screamed. I finally got to doses that did, in fact, knock her flat, but as they wore off a little she'd wake up howling. I asked a neurologist and a psychiatrist for help, but they were no more successful than I in finding a workable balance of medications. She tore out the feeding tubes we placed to give her some nutrition, and her weight dropped precipitously. Each morning I would find her gaunt decrepit figure in the bed, stark naked—even when tied down she always managed to get her clothes off—either in a drug-induced sleep or screaming.

Meanwhile, the insurance administrators nagged at me day after day to get her out of the hospital.

"She's stable. She has dementia." I could hear the masked irritation in the coordinator's voice.

"She doesn't. I know her. She didn't used to be like this."

"Well, this is her baseline now." *Stop being sentimental, thinking she'll get better, and get her out of there,* I could hear her thinking. "You're not doing any care in the hospital that she couldn't get in a nursing home."

"This is not her baseline," I repeated. "This is delirium tremens, and I'm sorry it's taking so long, but she needs hospital care until it's over."

I found myself, in the bleakness of the situation, taking absurd consolation from small triumphs over the insurance system. "Did I mention that she's in restraints?" I asked the coordinator brightly. "We can't send someone to a nursing home if they're restrained. I'm so sorry, but she'll have to stay."

Two and a half weeks passed, and finally the delirium tremens faded. She quieted at last.

Her body was spent from the weeks of struggle. As if she'd made enough noise in those weeks to last a lifetime, she became too quiet now, nodding and shaking her head to questions but rarely rousing the energy to speak. She was coherent, lucid enough as far as I could tell, but the light seemed to have gone out inside her. The psychiatrist agreed with me that she was probably depressed, but the antidepressants we tried didn't do much good. There seemed to be something empty inside her, some switch we couldn't turn back.

We transferred her to a nursing home. The coordinator's argument was fair, now; she needed food and strengthening, and the nursing home could do that as well as the hospital. I continued to hover over her closely. Physically she was well enough, but she was terribly weak. She spoke in single words on the rare occasions when she spoke at all. Her nutrition remained precarious; she swallowed well and had no trouble with the mechanics of eating, but her appetite was terrible.

"Ellie, you need to eat." The latest set of antidepressants and appetite stimulants were, like their predecessors, having no effect.

She nodded dumbly.

"And you need to do the physical therapy. Do you understand?

The physical therapists keep telling me they come and you won't work with them."

She hung her head.

"I know you don't like it, but you need that therapy to make you stronger. We have to get you strong enough to be able to go home."

George, her husband, had been sitting quietly beside her as I spoke, but stirred at the mention of home. "Ellie, you have to listen to her," he whispered. "Her dog won't eat," he added, addressing me but not taking his eyes off Ellie. "It's like they're doing it together, starving themselves. Her dog needs her."

"Rotten needs you," I said, in dead earnest. Only later would it occur to me to smile at this phrase.

She didn't seem to hear, and then she dissolved into wracking sobs.

She finally quieted, though she wouldn't talk to me about why she was crying, wouldn't say more than "I'm okay."

I pulled George aside. "Does she talk to you?" I asked.

"No."

"What was it like before, when you were at home? Before all this," I asked.

"Before she got sick, we would sit together in the house and spend hours and hours and days and not say anything. . . ." He said it dreamily, as if it were the happiest thing he could imagine. "I gave up the drink, you know," he said. Then he glanced up.

I had noticed this. He was always at her bedside when I came, and the smell of alcohol had slowly faded from him over the last few weeks.

"I knew she needed me to."

"That's wonderful of you."

"No. It's just what I needed to do."

"George . . . we have to make a decision, about whether to put a long-term feeding tube into her stomach. She's just not getting enough nutrition."

He nodded.

"I've tried to ask her whether it's something she wants," I went on. "But she won't answer. She said I should ask you."

"Does she need it?"

I struggled to find the right words. "George, if she's going to live, she needs food. More food than she's getting. So in that way, yes, she needs it. If she were stronger and better nourished, maybe she'd feel better, and want to eat. But maybe she's decided not to live, to let herself die. We'd be interfering with that, forcing food on her."

"I don't know," he said.

"Would she have wanted this, do you think? If we could have asked her, when she used to talk."

"Whatever you think is right, we'll do."

"I'm not sure I can answer that. It depends on what she would have wanted."

"I just want to get her home."

So the gastroenterologists placed a PEG tube, a little feeding tube into her stomach. Now at least she would get nutrition, she wasn't going to starve. There was no way to know if this was the right or wrong decision, choosing to force-feed her (not that it was exactly forcing, since she'd told me to ask her husband). It would depend on who she was and what she thought once she emerged from this strange silence—if she ever did.

Over the next two months her weight went up, and her nutritional parameters improved. But nothing much changed. I told her that if she were stronger she would be able to go home, but even that failed to light a spark.

I began plotting with George to get her home anyway. "Maybe she'll perk up, once she's there," we agreed hopefully. The physical therapists at the nursing home had stopped coming to see her, since she refused to work with them. She sat in bed most of the day, and George thought he could watch her as well at home as the nurses could here. We would get help for him to bathe her a few times a week, and help with other needs. Now we just had to teach him how to feed her through the PEG, and keep it clean.

It was the insurance company who told me, inadvertently, about the crisis.

"I'm just calling about Ellie—" said the coordinator's voice, briskly, on the phone. I was between patients, running a little late, and not thrilled to hear from her.

"Yes?"

"So you were going to have them work on training the family to do her PEG feeds, is that right?"

"They just started on Tuesday. I think it's going to take a little while to get everything in place. But I think it's going to work."

"You know about the husband, right?"

My medical assistant set another pile of charts on my desk, more work needing to be done, and I was getting testy.

"I know he's a chainsmoking recovering alcoholic and all that, is there something else I should know?" Even before I finished the sentence I registered the tone of her last question, and felt a sinking in my chest. "What is it, about her husband?"

"Well, as I understand it . . ." She stopped.

"What happened?"

"I don't know, but I understand that there was some kind of an event and he's at the Veteran's Administration hospital and they don't expect him to live."

"What?"

"He was found down by the medics. There was some kind of a devastating neurological event."

What strange words these are, when you think about them in human terms. "Found down," a term the medics use, somehow both technical and slang. "Devastating neurological event." An event. He suffered an event.

"I didn't know whether you knew. The nursing home has talked to the family about Ellie—there's nobody else close, but they found a cousin—and it sounds like they're planning to just leave her there until her coverage expires, and then she's got some backup with Medicare, so their plan is for her probably to stay there long-term—"

"Look—"

"Yes?"

"Stop."

"What?"

"I know George," I said. "We've worked together all this time. He's an actual person."

There was, finally, a meek pause on the other end of the line. "I'm sorry."

"I'm going to hang up now," I said evenly. "I'll see Ellie tonight. You and I will talk tomorrow."

"Okay," she said.

That evening I was at her bedside, unsure of what to say, not knowing even how much she knew or understood.

"Ellie."

She studied me with a clear eye. "Dr. Transue," she said. "It took me a minute to place you." She hadn't spoken my name since before she went into the hospital.

"Hi," I said gently.

"How's George?" she asked.

"He's—" I wasn't sure how to answer. "I talked to the doctors at the VA hospital a few hours ago, and he was about the same. Right now, I don't actually know."

She nodded. "Can you find out? I would like to know—"

"Sure. I can call and find out for you. . . ." To my surprise, she nodded expectantly and folded her hands as if to wait. "Do you want me to call right now?"

"There isn't a telephone in this room." She gestured around.

"I can call from the one in the hall. Wait just a minute, I'll be right back."

"His doctor says that he's about the same," I said when I returned. "His heart and lungs are stable but he isn't opening his eyes."

Very slowly, her eyes filled and the tears started streaming down her cheeks.

I sat on the bed, holding both her hands, wiping the tears away. "He loves you very much."

She nodded.

I stayed in close touch with the doctors at the VA over the following weeks. We arranged for her to visit him, a strange journey of one broken creature in a cabulance to the bedside of another. The VA nurses told me she was very quiet, that she sat at his bedside for two hours holding his hand, and kissed him quietly when it was time to go.

They called me two days later to tell me that he died. Peacefully, without ever waking up.

After the call I set my head down on my desk, heedless of my waiting patient, of the nervous shuffling of my medical assistant in the hallway. Grief overcame me. Partly at the loss of him, not a sophisticated man but a good and gentle one. Partly at the loss to her, of her companion of these fifteen years, the only person she had in the world . . . and, I realized, her only chance of getting to go home. Before her illness, she could have managed alone. But now? Yes, she'd been more alert in these last few weeks than she had been in months, but—could she live alone? I doubted she knew what day it was, much less how to care for herself, or manage an apartment. No, her last hope of leaving the nursing home had died with him.

Again, I was at her bedside, the small gray room that had become so familiar. The room where she would probably spend the rest of her days. I reached out my arms to her as I walked in, and she leaned against me.

"I want to get out of here. I just want to die." She began to cry, great wracking sobs. I took her hands in both of mine. "Your hands are cold," she murmured absently, through tears.

I thought of the call I got from the home earlier, that she was crying because of her husband. They wanted me to "give her something." Is there a pill for grief? I'd wanted to ask.

When she stopped crying she blew her nose, looked around for the wastebasket. "I'm working with his children on arrangements—"

I had forgotten he had children from a previous marriage.

"We've never gotten along much," she said, as if reading my thoughts. "But we'll do what we need to." She paused. "He'll be cremated," she added. "It's what he wanted."

We talked for a long time, and finally I got up to go. "I'll be back soon."

"I'll be here. Or who knows, maybe I'll be in the funny farm." Her eyes teared up again, but they had something of the old glint in them.

"Ellie. You're sad. It's normal to be sad when your husband dies. It's okay."

She nodded, still crying.

"Do you understand?"

"Yes."

There was a pause. I felt as if there should be something more that I could say.

"Is there anything else I can do for you?" It was an empty question, really. What could anyone do? To my surprise, she considered it carefully.

"I need a watch," she said at last. "I never know what time it is."

I looked around the room: there was not a clock in sight. It was pitch dark out, seven o'clock on a Seattle winter evening—it had been, I realized, just about a year since I first saw them, that snowy winter day. The sun sets early in Seattle in the winter, so the sky had been dark for hours. The room was dim, and the two other residents she shared it with were asleep. It could have been midnight.

I remembered that this was not the first time she'd mentioned a watch. A week or two ago, she'd said she couldn't read her old watch and she wanted to be able to know the time. Someone was supposed to bring a better one, she'd said. Clearly they hadn't.

"What kind of watch?" I found myself asking. I wondered what my teachers in medical school would have had to say about this situation.

"A Timex."

I nodded.

"One with big numbers, so I can see. I can't read the little ones."

"Okay."

"And a light. When you push the knob. So I can see it when it's dark."

I smiled. "You mean, like mine?"

She turned to look at my Timex with its big numbers and its backlight. "Yes."

"What color? Do you want a leather band, or metal?"

"Silver. Or gold. Yes—gold."

I brought the watch a few days later, just like mine except for its gold metallic band. At her bedside I adjusted the sizing to her tiny wrist. The face looked enormous beside her bony hand, but she could read it.

"Good," she said.

Her bed was scattered with papers, bills, insurance, documents needing signatures. I had not seen anything like this since she came here; in fact, she'd shown no interest in reading or in lifting a pen.

"Is there anything else you need?" I asked, with a little trepidation.

"I'd like a calendar. A little one. So I can know what day it is."

I nodded.

"And—" She thought a moment. "Chocolate. I want some chocolate. All they have here is pudding, and I can't stand pudding."

This was the first time she'd mentioned food since she went into the hospital.

"What kind of chocolate?" I asked, hoping she wouldn't come up with something prohibitively expensive, wondering where this was all going to end. And yet—she didn't seem as though she'd need much help for long.

"Kisses. Hershey's Kisses. Just a small bag."

"I'll bring them next time," I said, leaning over to kiss her cheek.

As I left she was leaning down, with a competent air, to arrange the papers on her lap.

10. FAMILY

As I thought about Ellie and George, my grandparents were also in my mind, another pair struggling in a very different way with illness and the possibility of separation. Those early years of my practice were an exploration of the interplay of love and loss, of grief and healing. Being a doctor was part of that: I was learning the role a primary care physician plays in people's lives, not passing briefly through as I had as a resident, but forging deeper, longer-term relationships. Being a daughter and a granddaughter was equally important, as I followed people I loved in the journey toward the end of life. The two roles enriched and informed each other.

My grandparents, given their dislike of doctors, would probably find this ironic. I never found out exactly what they had against the profession. I think it predated my father's cancer and everything that followed. My grandparents were fiercely independent and opinionated; maybe their dislike was rooted in a distrust of medicine's sometimes heavy-handed authority. Maybe my grandfather with his Ph.D. in mathematics had an academician's contempt for the pragmatic medical doctorate. They admitted to having liked only two doctors in their lives: one old friend who was also their personal physician for many years, and later, grudgingly, me.

My grandmother was French, born in Paris and raised in the French countryside. Her father was lost in World War I at the battle of Verdun; his body was never found, and her mother lived the rest of her long life as a half-widow, never fully convinced that he wouldn't return. Many years later my great-grandmother would travel around Europe tracking reports of men who had been war prisoners or lost their memories, not giving up hope that her husband might be out there somewhere. My grandmother was four years old when her father disappeared; from a young age she was no stranger to grief. There was no shortage of other losses, either. Decades later, looking at pictures from her childhood, she would point out to me all the people who died young: the aunt of tuberculosis, the uncles of the flu, the men of all ages killed at war. More of the people in her childhood pictures were dead by 1920 than alive.

My grandfather was from a small town in Pennsylvania, and went to Bordeaux on a scholarship in 1938 after he finished college. My grandmother's mother—left after the war with neither husband nor income—was supporting her small family by taking on boarders, mostly American students. My grandparents fell in love, married against the objections of both families ("They all told us it would never last," my grandparents told me nearly seventy years later), and returned to the United States. My grandfather was devastatingly handsome and charming, a classic rogue. They had three sons, of whom my father was the middle child, my grandmother's darling; she struggled to raise them in a land and culture far from her own, with little help or support. In the Second World War the family estate in France became a station of the French Resistance. My great-grandmother hid refugees from the Nazis while hosting and feeding the young German soldiers. My grandfather, meantime, was a civilian doing military support, and was dispatched to the Pacific to work on artillery design. My grandmother spent the war years living in cramped quarters in Pennsylvania with her in-laws and her sons, terrified for her husband and her family, and for the devastation of her country. Her oldest son was precocious and headstrong and the youngest was mildly developmentally delayed; she would later say my father was the easy one, but all three had powerful personalities.

After the war, things were easier. My grandfather taught mathematics at Kenyon and later at SUNY Binghamton. They made good friends—including the friend they would describe as the only doctor they'd ever liked. My grandmother taught French and gained a reputation for her wonderful cooking. The boys grew. They bought land on the coast of Maine and built a summer house there, where first their children and later we grandchildren spent our summers. My grandmother's later years—at least until my father became ill—were easier than her young ones. Still, there was a fierceness to her, a hard edge, that never softened, which I imagine was rooted in all her early hardship.

Though she would later be one of the most beloved people in my world, my relationship with my grandmother was rocky when I was young. In contrast to my grandfather, who doted on babies, my grandmother liked people to be clean and reasonable, and was impatient when her grandchildren failed to be either of these things. I knew she loved me, but whether she approved of me was much less clear.

My grandmother's house was a place of many and mysterious rules. The dinner table was a minefield that all of my generation approached with trepidation. Something as simple as passing a plate of bread around the table presented opportunities for error: Should you take your piece of bread off the plate and then take the plate itself, or the other way around? It depended on the genders and the relative ages and the degree of intimacy of the passer and passee, an unintelligible calculus. A sudden barrage of French, which we did not speak, was always the indicator that one of us children had done something wrong. My grandmother normally spoke English, though all her life (three quarters of it spent in America) she retained a thick French accent as a point of pride. Criticism, however, was always directed at us in her native tongue. We would all freeze, uncertain of the nature of the transgression: Had my lips left a crumb on the rim of my milk glass, which should always be clean? Had my brother used the communal butter knife on his bread instead of transferring the butter to his plate and then using his own butter knife? Our parents would eventually translate, and the meal would stumble on.

As the only girl among the grandchildren, I had perhaps the hardest time. She would push everyone to eat—another pitfall, since if all the food weren't eaten she'd declare you hadn't liked it, and if it were she'd bewail that there hadn't been enough. The only solution seemed to be to protest that the food was wonderful but I couldn't eat a morsel more, which was typically true. Heaven forbid, however, that I should use the word "full." It was fine for the boys, but I was told that in French the word for "full" was "pleine," and that if this were applied to cattle it could also mean "pregnant." Thus, by declaring myself satiated I had announced in the reverse-translated slang of a language that I did not speak that I was a pregnant cow. It was an unexpected avenue to rudeness for a small American child.

Even when she was speaking English, my grandmother maintained what I would later recognize as the French habit of understatement. If you had done something very well, she would say it wasn't bad. To say something was "nice" was actually lower praise. (I would later fall in love with much the same quality in medical language; I might have been hearing my grandmother's voice in dry turns of phrase like "It doesn't look good," our cover-all for terrible news. The worst medical catastrophe might elicit the description, "It's suboptimal.")

People were neatly labeled and critiqued: a neighbor was "reasonably pleasant but not pretty," or "friendly but not very bright." No praise went untempered; there was always a "but." As a child I thought this was mean; who cared if the neighbor was pretty, and was it impossible to say something simply kind? Likewise every experience was presented in balance: a concert was nice but the man in the next row was coughing. A sunny day was lovely but the night would be beastly hot. Even her smile turned down a little at the edges, as if too much pleasure would be unseemly.

As for me, I had done well in school but must remember that school was very easy at my age. I had won a piano contest, but I didn't play any pieces by composers she recognized. Accustomed to unbridled expressions of love and praise from my parents, I interpreted this "yes, but" construction as criticism. Only as an adult did I come to see it as a way of warding off ill luck. The world was a troubled place, and children ought not to be taught to expect too much of it. Pride was a grave evil and should not be encouraged. Hubris could be punished, even if it was only too great an enjoyment of a concert.

There were stories about my early childhood that were told over and over again, to my abject mortification. There was the time I visited my great-grandmother—my grandfather's mother—in the house my grandparents would later live in. I was three or four, already a tomboy but gussied into a pretty dress for the occasion. I went to play in the yard, rolling and digging in the dirt and grass, and returned to the house completely filthy, to everyone's horror. There was the time I got a child's rate on all-you-can-eat ice cream and proceeded to wolf down more than all the adults combined. Or the time we were at a restaurant with very slow service and I pulled the waiter over and lectured him that I was very hungry and needed my food right away. The message seemed clear enough: I had been a gauche, embarrassing little brat from the beginning.

Two things happened that completely changed my relationship with my grandparents. I grew up, and my father's mind began to fail. These both occurred so gradually and their time frames were so entwined that I don't know which was more important to our changing relationship. I went to college only a few hours' drive from my grandparents' home, and I would pop down for weekends with them that were a pure delight. They lived in a bright, quiet house in the Pennsylvania countryside, a perfect respite from the noise and bustle of New Haven. I would sleep in the luxury of a double bed in my own room, and wake up to the smell of bacon wafting up the stairs. Meals, which had been such a source of stress when I was a child negotiating foreign table manners, were now heaven on earth. Starved on bland dining-hall food, I treasured every morsel of my grandmother's fabulous French cooking. I helped in the kitchen, chopping nuts, spinning lettuce, and slicing radishes. She put her swollen feet up while I did the dishes, and after lunch, while both of them napped, I played the piano, having finally learned some Mozart and Chopin and Beethoven. She didn't comment on my playing, but she smiled; sometimes her smile didn't even have that little downturn around the edges.

We took walks to a nearby waterfall or along the Delaware River, talking about politics, music, art, books. Suddenly all the contentiousness of my childhood relationship with my grandmother was gone. There were no more tirades in French, which in the interim I had learned to speak. The measured phrases were still there—the grapefruits were good this year but the oranges were bitter; they'd reconnected with an old friend but his wife had Parkinson's—but they no longer struck me so darkly. I discovered, as other young people have, that this pair who I had always thought of only as grandparents had fascinating histories and lives.

My grandfather told me about working at the Princeton Institute for Advanced Study in the 1950s. Einstein's office was down the hall and my father and uncles used to beg nickels from him for the coke machine. NASA called my grandfather once to work on a project; he declined the job, and came home scoffing to my grandmother: "Those people are crazy! They think they can go to the *moon!*"

When I was very lucky, my grandmother would tell stories about France. These were convoluted tales that wove back through generations. They featured crazy relatives: the great-grandfather whose cat sat on his shoulder while he ate and plucked whatever morsels she wanted off his fork, another whose cat wandered up and down the table during meals and borrowed from everyone. Others detailed our famous antecedents: one of her great-grandfathers was on the survey vessel that was anchored at Milo when a farmer dug up the famous statue of Venus. According to family lore, her arms were lost as the French battled the Turks for possession of her (I checked this in the history books, which don't concur). My grandmother had a yellowed index card that detailed a precise lineage by which we were related to Joan of Arc—descended through Joan's brother and crossing marriage lines, but a connection nonetheless. There were antique soap operas of accidental pregnancies and forbidden marriages. There were stories of her girlhood, her grandmother's apartment in Paris, the estate in the small town where her grandfather was mayor. It was a magical world; I was entranced.

I am tempted to say that my grandmother had changed, but, of course, I was the one who was different. I had learned to listen, to come out of my world and into hers, where she was a willing hostess. Maybe now that I was grown, also, it was not so important to be vigilant against spoiling me, and maybe her priorities had shifted as well. My cousin had committed suicide, one uncle would always live a limited life, my father was ill, she and my grandfather were getting old. She lacked the comfort of religion; she had been raised Catholic, but had stopped believing as a young adult (except for a brief postpartum repentance after my father's birth, when she snuck a priest into the house in the night to secretly baptize him, knowing my lapsed-Episcopal grandfather would not approve). Maybe she had tired of the whole business of judging and disapproving, and reached a place where it was okay to simply enjoy the occasional gifts life offered: good food, a quiet house, or a nice granddaughter.

My grandfather was a quieter figure in the background of all this. He was a smiling, robust man, tall and silver-haired with a beatific grin. He had been wildly handsome in his youth and retained great elegance in age. If my grandmother plucked a negative perspective out of many things, my grandfather resolutely saw only the positive. Prior to my father's funeral I never saw him cry; I don't remember him even frowning. I adored him, a steadfast cheerful figure throughout my childhood, who favored me a little as the only granddaughter among four grandsons, and who always called me "pussycat." The phrase "unconditional love" has always brought my grandfather immediately to my mind. He was quiet in his contentedness, leaving most of the talking and all of the correspondence to my grandmother; I have hundreds of letters from her from over the years, each cosigned by him neatly at the bottom, "With love, your Grandfather." In a way, it was a metaphor for his presence in their house: ever present, a subject of great tenderness, but something of a postscript behind the force of my grandmother's personality.

Sometimes my father was there for the weekends I spent in Pennsylvania, during college and later medical school. He was living with his partner, who worked in Ohio for half of each year and in California the rest. My father's sexuality was something he didn't discuss with me directly; by the time I was mature and bold enough to ask openly for the full story of his experience, his mind was too far gone for him to answer. Arnold, his partner from soon after his split from my mother until the end of his life, cared for him throughout his illness with truly saintly devotion. My father moved back and forth with him between Ohio and California, but also spent several months each year with my grandparents in Pennsylvania or at their summer place in Maine. While my relationship with my grandparents was evolving into a close friendship, my father and I were simply and slowly reversing roles: I into an adult and he into a child. The slowness and the strange mental lapses, which became apparent when I was in college, had deepened by the time I was in medical school, to a point where he wandered in and out of an internal mental world, sometimes pinned by small details to reality but increasingly bizarre and paranoid.

He had strange fixations: the fear that I would burn myself on the stove, or the belief that I was having secret conversations in shadowy rooms in the house and lying about them. He exasperated my grandmother with the slowness of his movements and words—he spent the better part of dinner one day retelling the story of four-year-old me and the dirty dress, while the rest of us carried on a conversation interspersed with his phrases. Completing tasks for him was an embodiment of Zeno's paradox: he was always halfway done but never there. When he dried the dishes there were always a few left in the sink. If you reminded him, gently, he would dry a few more, but never all unless you hounded him to the last dish. Each of these traits, mild at first, got worse with each year that passed.

If the weekends I spent alone with my grandparents were simple bliss, the ones we shared with my father were much more complicated. There was his anguish, to begin with, at his increasingly frightening world, and at the dark messages it told him about me in particular (I sneaked, I lied). On top of that was his desire to take care of me, no less real for being painfully displaced (I could, by the time I finished medical school, be trusted with the stove). From my side there was irritation at his absurd solicitousness and a deeper pain and grief at what it represented, his failure to see or recognize me for what and who I was. In his world I was five or six years old. I knew better, but I couldn't completely suppress resentment at these belated attempts at nurturing from a parent who had been largely absent when I actually was young—the very thing he was probably trying to make up for. I struggled against the feeling that his imperviousness negated everything I had lived through and accomplished in the intervening twenty years.

My grandmother, for her part, cherished until near the end the belief that I could fix my father. In the early years, when his main symptoms were slowness and apathy, she believed I could fix him through the simple force of love; that if I were there to motivate him, if it were clear enough that I wanted him to be better, he would simply get better. I tried, although she always thought I could try harder; in any case, it made no difference. As time went on it became clear that something was more seriously wrong—this was the period of all the tests and evaluations, the dawn of the understanding that the radiation from his cancer had set in place an inexorable process of brain damage. When I started medical school, her hopes shifted. They didn't like doctors, but if I was nonetheless intent on becoming one, at least I would be in a position to cure my father.

Everyone in medicine struggles with this issue: Where do you draw the line between loved one and patient? When is it okay to give the people you love medical advice and when do you have to separate "caring about" from "caring for"? Some people are drawn to medicine because of the illness of a loved one, though I think this was not the case for me. If anything, my father's story was a disincentive from going into medicine, not a drive. It was clear to me from the beginning that I couldn't fix my father; even my emotional reactions to him were complex and cloudy, so how could I hope to have clear intellectual ones? I doubted that anyone could cure him, and I knew that even if someone could, it wouldn't be me. In any case I was vividly aware of disappointing my grandmother.

When it became clear that neither my doctoring nor anyone else's had a cure in store, she wished that I would nurse him. She didn't directly ask me to; the suggestions were more oblique. *Aren't there good hospitals in California, or Ohio? Do you think about taking time off? You're young, you can always go back to training later. He's so much happier when he sees you, he would be so much better if you were there.* And in its starkest form: *If I die, I don't want him to be alone.*

He was not, of course, alone. Arnold, his partner, tended him, made sure he got the best possible medical care, kept him at home as long as humanly possible and, when that was no longer safe, found residential care for him. By the time I finished my medical residency my father was in a nursing home, where Arnold visited him daily. Perhaps my grandmother would have focused less on me if there had been a wife instead of another man taking care of him, though I don't know. As it was, though she acknowledged and was profoundly grateful for everything Arnold did, she thought it should have been me.

We never had the conversation openly; I never said, I love my father but I won't give up my life for him, partly because he wouldn't have wanted me to, partly because he didn't build the kind of relationship with me that makes a person willing to give up everything. I didn't say, I might put off my career to move here and take care of you if you needed it, but I can't, or I won't, do it for him. I did promise that I would always visit him, that once she was gone I would bake him the cookies that she had always made, that he would not feel abandoned by his flesh and blood. It was an imperfect answer, but she accepted it. Though there was always some reproach in my grandmother's discussions with me about my father, it didn't cloud my relationship with her. In fact, she and I were probably closer than we would have been if he were well. The care we took to stay in touch, our heightened solicitousness and attention for each other, was partly driven by his illness. In a different world, he might have been there to take care of both of us; instead, we took care of each other. I treasured that, even while feeling painfully guilty, on his account and on hers, for not doing what she wanted me to do.

Once I moved to Seattle for residency I saw my grandparents less. I visited when I could, popping out for weekends on the red-eye, my sleep deprivation matching the limited energy of their age. I had realized some time before that I would never write the letters to them that I intended (my grandmother was a prolific correspondent, while my father, even before his illness, could hardly get a letter in the mail; I fell somewhere in between), and when I started medical school I resolved instead to call them every weekend. I kept to this plan religiously, although after some years a chance comment by my grandmother revealed that I called every Sunday night just before nine, the latest time at which they considered it polite to call. Apparently my habit of procrastination had run up against my resolution to call on the weekend and arrived at the Sunday-night solution. My grandmother was not as comfortable with the phone as with mail, and for the first year or two the conversations were awkward. My grandparents had their generation's view of telephones—they were used to letting people know when someone died—so once we'd established that everyone was okay and I was just calling to say hello, they ended the conversation. Finally, however, they relaxed. By the time I started practice we had been having weekly conversations for eight years, and my grandmother would sometimes tell me stories over the phone, a radical departure for her. They always used their speaker phone, although it had

terrible voice quality, and every conversation with them was peppered with static. My grandmother and I would talk, and just as we
were about to hang up, my grandfather—just as in their letters—would
lean into the phone and say, "Love you, pussycat," before hanging up
the receiver.

When I started practice, my grandparents were in their late eighties
and were beginning to struggle with their health. The presence of
doctors in their lives, so long averted, had become a necessary evil.
My grandfather had a small stroke. My grandmother developed re-
current intestinal bleeding. Each of them spent a little time in the
hospital, during which it became clear how much the two depended
on each other, how completely they had segregated their household
roles. My grandfather had trouble writing after his stroke, and it
emerged that my grandmother had never written a check. My grandfather barely knew how to use the toaster. They still lived alone in the
house in the countryside, and with each illness the younger generations held our breaths to see if they would still be able to keep the
household going. We murmured in hushed tones about nursing
homes, imagining in horror how my grandmother, with her rigid
standards and inflexible tastes, would manage outside her house—the
table had to be set and the beds made just so, not to mention how
strongly she felt about good food, and how much she disliked the in-
terference of other people.

Each time things seemed to be in crisis, however, my grandparents somehow righted themselves. They found a housekeeper who
met my grandmother's standards. When my grandmother was too
weak to do the laundry she sat beside the machine and showed my
grandfather what to sort into which pile, which detergent to use, and
which button to press. Meantime, declaring him to be too "gaga"
since the stroke to handle the accounts ("gaga," a benign version of
senility, was a favorite word: *She's healthy but she's getting very gaga*, or
He's weak but not at all gaga; interestingly, she never used the word

to describe my father) she took over the family finances with a vengeance. With the same determination with which they had faced two wars, the disabilities of two sons, the death of a grandson, and countless other struggles through the years, they stared down the difficulties of age.

Each week when I talked to them it seemed that there had been another death. Not only were their friends dying, but the next generation—old students, younger friends and protegés—were dying, too. They were meticulous in their reporting of the details: whether it had been at home, whether slow or fast, whether there had been pain. "He was lucky; it was quick, and he was home." They were mostly philosophical about the losses, and about the knowledge that their own deaths would come. "The time comes for us all. We've lived well. Perhaps it's better not to live so long." I think they grieved the passing of their generation more than the individuals they lost; the world they had known was disappearing. It was a sort of reverse Brigadoon; everyone else had faded into the mists of the past, and here they were, still moving into an unknown future.

Even as my roots grew deeper in Seattle, my heart was divided. A warm, anxious piece of my self was in Pennsylvania, and a tender, troubled part in California. I carried these worries and cares with me to the office, just as I carried the grief of my patients' losses home. As I watched my grandparents muse over their lives I thought about my patients, and tried more deeply to imagine them in the full context of their lives. How could I help someone feel at the end that they had lived well, and to count the manner of their death as "lucky"? What comfort could I offer to families whose loved ones were going through what my father was going through? For myself, as I struggled to carry the grief of losing patients, I wondered also how to reconcile my grandparents' matter-of-fact approach to death with my own anguish at the thought of losing them.

As I puzzled over how to connect my life as a doctor to my grandparents' lessons about grief and loss, they remained dry on the subject of doctoring. "Your grandfather has to go in tomorrow for a blood test for his warfarin," my grandmother said one Sunday night at the end of our weekly conversation. She had finally stopped calling his medication rat poison. "Personally, I think it's all a scam for the doctors to make money. That's how they operate, you know.

"Have a good week," she added. "Save some lives."

"Love you, pussycat," my grandfather said.

"I love you, too," I said.

LAUGHTER AND LOSS

11. THE PEGGY AFTERNOON

Medicine, of course, also has its light moments. Helping people to stay healthy is a cheerful undertaking, and is a large part of what we do. Best of all, the day-to-day life of doctoring can frequently be quite funny—often, for better or worse, at my own expense.

The most embarrassing moments of my medical career comprise, sadly, neither a short nor a trivial list. Many of them revolve around certain themes: the trick of memory by which I can remember almost anything about people (their pets, their grandchildren, their hobbies) except their names, even after a relatively long and close acquaintance. The peculiar form of dyslexia that causes me to be completely incapable of knowing which of my patients is in which of my two exam rooms, even if I have just come out of one, so that I am always bursting in on the wrong person unannounced, and then having to apologetically back out again. Then there was the time that I had an almost hour-long consultation with a new patient, reviewing her background in full detail, not realizing until she stood to leave and leaned toward me saying, "Don't you love Kirsten's baby? She's so beautiful!"—that she was someone I already knew. We had chatted with each other at some length at my friend's wedding the year before, and, indeed, she'd described then some of the life history we'd reviewed this morning.

The most mortifying story to date, however, would surely have to be the Peggy afternoon.

Peggy Anderson was a patient of mine who was prone to chest pain and anxiety, and who had just spent a few days in the hospital having her heart evaluated. Everything checked out fine, and on the morning in question she was discharged from the hospital and headed, I believed, home to her house on the Olympic Peninsula, several hours away from Seattle. On the way, however, she called and left a message with my medical assistant saying that her grandson had just been diagnosed with meningitis, and she was wondering whether she needed to be tested or treated. She'd seen him before her hospitalization; would any of the tests we'd done there show if there was a problem?

I got the message and asked my medical assistant to call her back and get more information, specifically about what kind of meningitis the child had, and when and how she had been exposed to him. Without that, I couldn't tell what she should do. The tests we'd done in the hospital probably wouldn't be relevant, since they were mostly on her heart. My medical assistant called, got her answering machine, and left a message for her to call back.

An hour or so later, my receptionist came to the medical assistant and let her know that Peggy was calling back. The medical assistant picked up the call and explained, "We need to have a little more information before we can tell you what to do."

"I'm just calling about the results," Peggy said.

"We don't have any results," my medical assistant said. "We need to have more information."

"But what does the test tell us?"

"Well, there are different kinds of tests, but before we talk about that I need to know more about the exposure."

"Exposure?"

"We don't know if you need to worry about meningitis until we know more about the exposure."

"I'm not worrying about meningitis, all I want is the result."

"Well, I'm glad you're not worried, but the doctor needs more information."

At this point the connection abruptly cut out. My medical assistant tried to return the call, got the answering machine again, said she was sorry about the confusion over the test results, but could she please call back as soon as possible.

A few minutes later the receptionist brought back another message, explaining that Peggy had called back from a pay phone, that she was not actually at home but on her way to spend the weekend in Oregon. She left her cell phone number, but noted it was behaving erratically in the area she was in. She said she should have better coverage later.

Half an hour later Peggy called again.

"We don't have any test results," my medical assistant said.

"I just want to know if I should be worried, if I should be taking anything."

"I thought you weren't worried."

"Well, I don't know. I try not to worry. But isn't meningitis dangerous?"

"It can be. It depends on what kind it is. Do you know if his meningitis is bacterial, or viral? It's very important."

"I don't know. I can call his mother and try to find out."

"That would be great."

"I'll call you as soon as I know."

Another half hour, and she called back again. "I think I've got it all straightened out."

"Oh, good."

"The phone wasn't working."

"I understand. Have you found out what kind of meningitis it was?"

"Was there meningitis on my tests?"

"We haven't done these particular tests. We're just trying to get the information."

"I just want to know about the tests."

"We haven't done them yet."

"But your message said you had, and I should call."

"No, the message said we needed to talk to you, so we could ask you some questions."

"But I thought it was about the tests I had last week."

"The doctor didn't test for meningitis in the hospital."

"Not the hospital. The clinic. I want the results of the tests I had in clinic."

"But you didn't have any tests in clinic, they were all in the hospital."

"What hospital?" she asked.

My medical assistant, alarmed, put her on hold and brought this news back to me. I was tending to a young woman who had just fainted after getting a shot, and I didn't feel comfortable leaving the room, so my medical assistant and I conferred in a whisper. "She doesn't remember being in the hospital."

"She doesn't remember being in the hospital?" I repeated.

She shook her head solemnly.

"But she just left this morning," I said, thinking aloud. "That doesn't make any sense. But you said she seemed confused. . . . Is it possible that she's delirious? Ask her if she has a fever. Or a headache."

She came back a moment later. "She has a little bit of a headache. She doesn't think she has a fever, but she isn't sure."

"Is she feeling sick? Does she have a rash?"

"She says she's okay and she just wants her test results."

"I'll call her back as soon as I can. Tell her if she starts to feel even a little bit sick she needs to go to the nearest ER for an evaluation. And we'll need to have her come in as soon as she gets back from Oregon."

"She said okay, but she sounded pretty confused."

Only a moment later she called again, to ask what these tests were that we were leaving her messages about. My medical assistant explained, once again, that we hadn't yet done any tests. Peggy explained that she understood that, but she didn't understand why we were leaving messages about confusion about tests when there hadn't been any tests. In any case, she had learned that her nephew had viral meningitis, not bacterial. She wasn't able to remember when she had last seen him—a week ago, or maybe two? Her memory was just appalling, she complained. It seemed to be getting worse by the minute.

"More problems with her memory?" I said when my medical assistant relayed this. "Ask her again about the hospital."

Certainly, my assistant relayed, she remembered being in the hospital that morning. "She doesn't remember telling me she didn't!"

"But it was just a minute ago!"

"She says she couldn't have been talking to me a minute ago, she doesn't have a cell phone and she just got home."

"I thought she was on the cell phone, and that she wasn't at home, she was in Oregon."

"She says she's at home."

At this moment the receptionist poked her head in, to say that Peggy was calling back on the other line.

It took some time to piece together (or more accurately, to piece apart) the various conversations with both Peggys, the one from the hospital with the grandson, and the other one, who truly had just been returning a call we'd made the day before about some tests she'd done in clinic. It took more time yet to persuade them both that neither they nor we had meningitis, or any other dangerous cause of delirium.

Luckily they both forgave us. Indeed, they both thought the whole incident was hysterical, once all was finally explained. I, for my part, learned a valuable lesson, or rather two: a simple one on the importance of last names and clear identities, and a deeper principle, that when something doesn't seem to add up it probably really doesn't. In the future, before suspecting someone else of bizarre behavior, I would first examine my own.

12. MARGARET

As always, the funny moments were interspersed with sad ones. The first time I met Margaret Wilson, I asked about the strange glass locket she had around her neck. It was a square box with a small fragment of something slate-gray in it. I suspected it had a story—a piece of rock from the family farm, or in another vein, a mystical magnet or crystal. I was prepared for the off chance that it might be a bit of her husband's ashes.

She held it up. "This? You want to know about this?"

"Yes," I said, less sure now.

"This is the bullet they took out of my grandson's back at his autopsy."

Then she began to cry.

She had ten children. Eleven pregnancies, one stillbirth. "There's one I don't talk to so maybe that's nine." Otherwise she'd been very healthy. She had worked doing all kinds of things—housekeeping, office work, gardening—anything to keep food in the children's mouths. "I lost my husband young. We did what we had to. I don't know if I was a good mother, but I kept them clothed and fed."

"Of course, you were a good mother," I said. "Just to have survived, you had to be."

I'd known her for about a year when she came in coughing up blood. Just a little blood, but still. I pressed: Had she had a recent cold? Sinus trouble? Nothing she could remember.

Coughing up blood is a symptom that scares people. Young non-smokers with bronchitis will cough up a spot of blood and come in, afraid they have cancer. Often enough it's just a viral infection, or a bloody nose. But Margaret wasn't young, and she'd smoked, though she quit years ago.

Her lungs sounded fine. "I'd like to get a CT scan, to have a closer look."

"But you haven't even done a chest X-ray."

It was her voice more than her words that carried the sudden note of fear. I always watch for this, the moment when a patient becomes afraid. Some of them come in scared, even over something that seems trivial to a medically experienced eye. You can tell at a glance that some skin lesions aren't cancerous, but it takes a special kind of reassurance to calm someone who is seized with the belief that they're going to die.

For other people fear comes later, with the utterance of certain words: "spot," "tumor," "biopsy." You never know what will trigger it: I had a patient once who went ashen at being told she had a kidney infection. Her mother had died of kidney failure, an entirely different beast, but the word "kidney" was enough. So you have to watch for fear, even when you don't expect it. Likewise the expected shocking words—"cancer," "death"—leave some unfazed. You can never tell which word or moment will bring someone into abrupt confrontation with her mortality.

With Margaret, the only time I saw her flinch was when I said "CT."

Silently I confronted her fears, and mine. She was right, in fact, that jumping right to the CT scan reflected my concern that this was something serious. We could get an X-ray first, but if it was fine I wouldn't trust it; I'd get a CT to look more closely. On the other hand, if the X-ray was abnormal I'd get the CT to clarify the problem. We were headed to the scan either way.

"A regular X-ray won't give us the information we need. We need to get the CT."

"Okay." Her eyes met mine, warily.

The scan showed a mass in her lungs, small but spiky—worrisome looking. A series of additional tests followed. The hospital's fancy new PET scanner showed that the little mass was consuming too much sugar, using too much energy. It was trying too hard, growing too fast to be benign.

"I'm so sorry, Margaret, but all the signs are pointing toward it being cancer. It needs to come out."

This time she didn't even wince. "Whatever we need to do."

The surgery went smoothly. The mass was a lung cancer, but it was small and the surgeon felt confident he had gotten it all. Margaret was drugged pretty deeply on pain medication for a couple of days, cheerful but only half coherent on my daily visits.

Her oldest daughter, Jill, called me about four days after the surgery.

"How are you doing with all this?" I asked.

"Well, I'm—" Her voice choked up, but I didn't expect what she said next. "I have to say I'm pretty disappointed in you."

My stomach sank as if I had been hit. "I'm sorry?"

"She's been in the hospital all this time and you haven't even been to see her. . . ."

Understanding dawned suddenly. "Jill, I see her every day."

A pause. "You do?"

"She's been on a lot of drugs," I said. "Has she said anything else to make you think she was confused?"

"She was talking to my father," she admitted softly. "He died forty years ago. That was one of the reasons I wanted to talk to you. Dr. Transue, I'm sorry, I didn't mean to—"

"No, no," I said. "It's fine. I'm sorry, I should have been in touch with you all along. But I'm glad we're talking now, and next time you're mad at me, call sooner. Now, about her pain medications . . ."

In another few days her thinking had cleared, and her surgical wounds were beginning to heal. We transferred her to a nursing home where she could get physical therapy and wound care until she was strong enough to go home.

A few days after the move I found her with Jill, looking out the window and talking quietly. "How are you doing?" I asked.

She shrugged and ran her fingers through her hair. "I've come this far; I've had worse times than this. I've not had an easy life. But my children are all grown and it doesn't matter so much what happens to me now."

I nodded. "That's fair enough. Still, I think what's going to happen now is that you're going to heal and feel better—"

I listened to her lungs and heart. I had a feeling more conversation was coming, but I didn't want to rush it.

"I think you're doing beautifully," I said.

"I'm doing okay," she said. "I'm not young. It takes an old body time to heal. Not that age is everything. . . ."

She paused significantly, and I wondered if she was thinking about the grandson she lost to violence, the baby born dead, the husband whose death I've never dared ask about. I glanced at Jill. She was straightening some of Margaret's things, and didn't look at me.

"My husband was young, you know," Margaret said.

I waited for her to say more, but when she didn't, I asked. "How did he die?"

"Heart failure, they said. I didn't allow an autopsy, so we'll never really know. I didn't think he'd want it."

She sighed, as if she wished now she had made a different choice. How different a person she must have been, forty years ago.

"He'd never had trouble with his heart. He thought he had the flu. He didn't feel well for a week or two, and then his legs started blowing up and he couldn't breathe. He went in and they gave him a sedative and put a tube down his throat, right then.

"After a couple of days they said they thought he was stronger, that they could let him wake up and he would breathe on his own. So they stopped the sedative and they took out the tube and he died. It was only a few minutes."

She frowned. "Or maybe it was hours. I don't remember."

We were interrupted by the woman in the next bed, who was flailing against the divider curtain between her bed and Margaret's.

"Do you need to get out?" I poked my head around to her side of the curtain.

She was completely naked. "No, I don't need to get out. I was just trying to get to that side of the bed so I could get my clothes—"

I reached for one of the two sweaters lying on the bed.

"Not that one, the blue one. That's the one I always wear to my treatments."

What kind of treatments? I wondered. Or perhaps did she just imagine that she was going somewhere? She seemed confused.

This question was answered as a handsome young medic walked into the room, nodded to acknowledge me and Margaret, then reached for the other woman's curtain.

I started to warn him. "She's not dressed—" I wasn't quick enough. He stuck his head into her enclosure and drew back suddenly. "I'll just leave you alone a moment more," he told her through the cloth, and left the room.

I turned back to Margaret. "How long am I going to be in here?" she asked me quietly, glancing around the room.

"As long as it takes for your strength to build up so you'll be okay at home."

"Is my insurance going to kick me out?"

There was a time when this question would have shocked me. More shocking still was that the answer might be "yes." I've learned not to be shy in discussing unpleasant truths, about money as well as health.

"Sooner or later your insurance will have something to say about it. When you're well enough to be at home, or not making progress in the therapy here, they'll make some noise. They've got their rules. But honestly, I think before they have a chance to say anything you'll be chomping at the bit to get out of here. Home to your own food and your own bed and peace and quiet."

There was an explosion of noise from the hallway as a loaded tray fell off a meal cart. The sound of clanking metal and breaking china echoed through the halls. "Peace and quiet?" she asked. I tried to suppress a grin.

At that moment another wild flailing came from behind the neighbor's curtain, as if a bird were tangled in it.

"Do you need help?" I called, careful to respect her privacy this time.

"I just need to get out!"

She sounded irritated, as if she hadn't chided me a minute ago for offering this very thing. I drew back the curtain for her. A moment later, the handsome young medic returned and wheeled her away.

"We were talking about when your husband died," I said to Margaret, as the neighbor's wheelchair disappeared.

She nodded.

"How old were your children then?"

"The youngest was born six weeks later. Harold. You met him when I was in the hospital, I think? He was born when his father was six weeks in the grave.

"The oldest was seventeen. You."

She nodded at Jill, who had begun combing Margaret's fine gray hair as we talked, weaving it into a long thin braid on the top of her head.

"I didn't have any money. I took what little I had from the life insurance after I buried him, and made a down payment sight unseen on a house in Seattle. We were living near Los Angeles then; it was cheaper here. I put the kids in the wagon and drove up here to a house I'd never seen.

"I'd never owned a house before. I was naive. I didn't know much about it. I got insurance but it turned out it was only—what do you call it? Mortgage insurance."

Her daughter finished the braid and moved away, fluffing pillows for a third patient across the room, offering to bring her water. As if she didn't want to listen.

"I was having an addition put on the house, and I had to get an extra loan for that. But that part wasn't insured because it wasn't finished yet. I went away for the weekend, and there was a fire and the house burned down."

She said it matter of factly, without emotion.

"So. The mortgage insurance paid the bank but there was the money I borrowed for the addition, and there we were again, the eleven of us, with nothing."

Jill drifted back. "We made it work." I took note for the first time of her solid body in a nurse's uniform.

Margaret nodded slowly. "We did."

"Funny," she added a moment later. "Everyone in my family had heart attacks. So I always assumed, you know, that it would be the heart that would get me. Not cancer."

"It hasn't got you," I reminded her softly.

"Well, we'll see. Either way, I've lived a good life."

This didn't seem like a point that I should argue with.

"I understand you saw my friend Alice yesterday. She's written me a note every day since I've been in the hospital.

"She writes long letters. Types them. She'll send a card with a few words printed on it and then she'll have filled the whole thing front and back with typing, and attached another page or two besides. And she sends jokes, you know, bits from the newspaper, and stories.

"She's lonely. She only has two children."

What poverty that must seem—just two!—to someone who carried ten!

Alice, for her part, had mentioned her notes in my office yesterday. "I have trouble thinking of things to say, to these old people," she'd said, rubbing her arthritic hands. "You have to be careful, to pick the jokes and things that are appropriate!"

I smiled at the thought of these two old friends, quietly and tenderly pitying each other.

As predicted, Margaret's energy soon returned and she was raring to get out. We picked a day for discharge, but on the chosen morning her daughter called to ask if we could delay a little. "Either way is fine with me," I said. "If she wants to stay, she can stay."

"I think she'd like to have another day," Jill said.

"That's fine."

I arrived at the nursing home a few hours later to discover the situation was more complicated. Margaret was screaming into her phone.

"I'll take a cab home if no one will take me. It's my own house, dammit! You can't keep me out of there."

I flinched.

But the telephone was still pressed to her ear, and suddenly her tone softened. "Now, Jill—," chastened. "I only meant—," then another pause. "I know you would." A deep sigh. "Oh dear, I didn't mean for you to be upset—"

"Do you want me to talk to her?" I whispered. She nodded and handed me the phone.

"Jill, I'm just here with your mother, and she's just been saying how incredibly helpful you've been through all of this." I was improvising a little.

Across the line, Jill sniffled.

"But I think she's pretty anxious to go home."

Margaret rolled her eyes at me.

The report from the pathologists was good. The spot was small and well contained, though the cells were a kind that could grow fast. The lymph nodes were free of cancer cells. It looked like we had it all.

She saw me frequently while her surgical wounds were healing and her strength was building up. There were a lot of details to talk about: her appetite, her activity, her bowels, her pain.

On her third or fourth visit as she stood to go she cleared her throat.

"Yes?"

"Um. I was talking to the oncologist, the one who said it was all gone, that we didn't need to do anything more."

I wasn't sure where this was going. "Yes."

"And . . . well, I guess you and my surgeon saved my life. You found it. He took it out."

I nodded.

"I guess—I guess I should say thank you."

She looked acutely uncomfortable. More uncomfortable in the face of gratitude than in discussing her husband's death or her house burning down.

"Margaret, you're welcome. But don't sweat it, all right?"

"Thanks." She grinned, and looked relieved.

As she walked away I noticed that she wasn't wearing the necklace, the one with the bullet.

13. AFTERNOON OFF

It was one of the first, glorious days of spring, when the temperature finally shifts from crisp to warm. I was working only half a day, but nothing went right. Everything seemed out of synch. It was like trying to play a piece on the piano that you know perfectly well and have played a thousand times before, only this time it refuses to come out of your fingers. The more you struggle the more it doesn't work.

To begin with, my schedule was too crowded. Then we had to squeeze someone in with an emergency. Everybody seemed to have a couple of extra "little" questions they just wanted to deal with "while I'm here." *Do you deal with the other professionals in your life this way?* I wanted to ask. *Do you schedule time with your accountant to do your taxes and then ask them to rearrange your investments, "since I'm here anyway?"*

It was only a half day, so even running late I would have the afternoon to myself. As I was sifting through my piles of paperwork, an hour after I meant to leave, my medical assistant popped her head in. "Michelle from scheduling just called to say that she's sorry. Somehow there was a mix-up and the person who was supposed to do our reminder calls for today forgot and didn't do them."

I looked up at her. "Everybody came anyway, and it was a catastrophe."

"Yes, well, I told her it had all worked out."

"Maybe we should have someone call and remind them they don't have to come."

"Remind them how sunny it is outside."

"Ask them if they've called their children, parents, grandparents, or grandchildren lately. Ask them whether on their deathbeds they're going to look back and be glad they came to the doctor today."

We were both in giggles now.

"Okay, really, I have to get out of here—" I only had one free afternoon a week, and I guarded it like a treasure.

I changed into shorts and started walking toward downtown. My big agenda item for the afternoon was to go to a lighting store downtown and replace a broken halogen bulb. Walking down the street in my T-shirt, shorts, and sandals, I saw one of my patients coming toward me on the sidewalk. I'd seen her outside work before: she worked at a flower shop near my house. At first, I had worried she might launch into a detailed discussion of her medical issues among the roses and gladiolas. I've never completely gotten over a bad experience some years ago with an uninhibited patient who explained his strange rectal symptoms at great length in the grocery store. This woman, however, was always pleasant and professional.

She smiled at me brightly as we passed by each other.

"That thing you gave me," she said. "It worked!"

"That's great!" I said. I couldn't for the life of me remember what I had last given her, or why.

"It worked great. Right away."

"I'm so glad."

"Take care," she said, and continued on her way.

That wasn't so bad. Please, though, I thought to myself as I continued walking. Can't I just be myself for the rest of the day, instead of Dr. Transue?

The day was a glorious one, and by the time I reached downtown my worries were softening under the bright sun and the pleasure of exercise.

I walked up to the repairs counter. "I was just hoping you had another of these bulbs—" I reached into my bag for the broken fragment.

"Hey, I was meaning to call you!"

I looked up and, of course, she was one of my patients. Also, of course, I couldn't remember her name.

Luckily she had a name tag. I sneaked a glance at it surreptitiously. Sally. Of course. Sally Watson.

"I've been thinking for two weeks that I should call you, and I was thinking today I was finally going to do it."

"Why?" I asked weakly, against my better judgment.

"I've been having this chest pain."

Please tell me this is a joke.

"Chest pain?"

"Right here."

She bared her left breast slightly, there at the counter.

"Ah. Are you . . . Are you having it now?" I asked, with great trepidation.

She thought for a second. "Yes!"

I was a little dizzy. *This isn't happening. I just want my bulb.*

"Is it sharp?"

"It's really sharp." She paused. "It's worse when I take a deep breath. See?"

She took a couple of deep breaths, although I couldn't really see anything.

"Ummm . . ." What was I supposed to say? Please pick up the phone, dial my office, and ask to speak to the person covering for me?

Okay, Em, step up to the plate.

"Are you short of breath with it at all?"

"Short of breath?" She thought for a moment. "No, not really."

"Has it gotten any worse over the last two weeks?"

"No. It just hasn't gone away."

"Is it worse when you exert yourself?" A good general screening question for heart pain.

"Actually it's worse when I'm resting."

"Have you had any swelling in either of your legs, and have you been on any long car or airplane trips lately?" These questions were aimed at blood clots, another dangerous cause of sharp chest pain.

"No."

Thank goodness, I thought. No warning signs for anything terrible, anything that couldn't safely wait a day or two. "Call my office and make an appointment for tomorrow."

"Oh, okay."

I gave her the number.

"Thanks." She wrote it down. "Well, okay, then, thanks. . . ." She smiled, as if expecting me to walk away.

"Um . . . Do you think you could help me find this lightbulb?"

We found the bulb, and I offered her a charge card. It didn't have my photograph.

"Can I see some ID?" she asked, without irony.

I opened my mouth to comment, then closed it, and pulled out my driver's license, savoring the pretense of anonymity.

14. CALIFORNIA POPPIES AND BLEEDING HEARTS

As my practice settled into a routine, there was still turmoil going on in my family. On an early spring morning, I knelt in my garden planting plants. Columbine and clematis, bleeding hearts and California poppies. Irises and lilies of the valley, strawberries and hyacinths and honeysuckle.

A thousand miles away in California, my father was waiting to have most of his teeth pulled out, and I was in Seattle planting flowers. California poppies, bleeding hearts.

I dug the way he taught me to dig, as a child of four or five, when my parents still lived together. I filled the little holes with water, placed the seedlings into holes, tucked dirt neatly around the stems. I remembered with the kinesthesia of childhood the particular feel, the unique consistency of soaked dirt pressed into the roots of a young plant, the dirt itself supple, seemingly alive. I watered the way he taught me, a light spray, not too much, but long enough to soak through all the layers of the surrounding earth. My house is the first I've ever owned; the last garden I had was the one he and my mother planted.

I knelt, planting plants and knowing I should be with my father. I would go soon; I had to see him one more time while he still had his teeth. He was too confused to handle dentures, and his teeth were infected and breaking; he ground the fragments painfully against each other, making a startling, percussive noise. I understood that they needed to come out, but still I dreaded it. Even without his knowing my name, and with his unfocussed eyes that didn't seem quite the color they used to be, still there was a sometimes a glimmer of a smile, some twitch of mouth in which I could see the father I once knew. Without his teeth, I was terrified there would be nothing left to recognize.

It was hard for me to tell, in relation to my father, what I was talking myself into and what I was talking myself out of at any given moment. I could say: My father would want me to be here planting things, giving life to the little seedlings. I noticed that every one of the flowers I had carefully selected and brought home was a kind that he loved. As my thoughts wandered, I moved on to a new section of the yard and began planting roses. Roses and more roses, his very favorite. Growing roots in the life I was building as the adult he never knew. He would want me to be doing this, not weeping on an airplane flying to or back from visiting the faint shadow of himself. I could tell myself this, and probably it was true.

I could also say that it didn't matter whether I went, that he didn't remember I had been there five minutes after I was gone. I could say, that for every afternoon I spend in the locked-in courtyard of his nursing home trying to talk or not trying to talk, or trying or not trying to feed him, or showing him picture-books, I lost a little more of him. A little more of the memory of planting roses faded, another cloudy layer of sorrow was taped over an already scant collection of memories of a father whom I loved, but who hadn't been around much even when he was healthy and I was young.

Each of these things was true, though terrible. Still, I needed to go. Partly for my grandmother, who felt better when I went, but it was more than that. There was some simmering restlessness that could be answered only by going. Here again (talking myself into, talking myself out of), I didn't know if this was just a cheap assuagement of guilt, a way of pretending I had done something when really I hadn't and perhaps I couldn't. A painful, pointless show, walking over coals. Why did I go at all, if it did neither of us any good? If it did, then why didn't I go more often? Either way there were thick, uneasy compromises.

I planted, and pondered.

Arnold had managed to keep my father at home for an amazingly long time. Finally, though, during my third year of residency, he became too sick to manage without full-time nursing care. He went to a specialized dementia nursing home very close to their old house, where friends could take him walking in the familiar neighborhood. The staff were kind, and the facility was pretty and clean. It was everything one could hope for in such a place, although, of course, such a place in itself isn't exactly what one hopes for.

The nursing home was called Arbor House. It was an unassuming building on a residential street, painted pale yellow. A iron fence ran around it, just a little too high to climb, with a small mechanical gate and a walled-in garden. Apart from the fence, there was nothing to distinguish it from the surrounding buildings. A sign at the entrance directed visitors to push a button on a nearby fencepost to open the gate. All facilities for people with dementia have some variation on this: a one-way valve for functioning minds.

Chris met my father there for the first time, when we were residents. My father had only recently moved in. We found him in the big living room, with chairs arranged in concentric half-circles around a television. He didn't look up, so I went over and took his hand.

"Oh," he said. "Oh." He smiled at me, then turned to Chris in puzzlement.

"This is my friend," I said.

"It's nice to meet you, Mr. Transue," Chris said formally, and they shook hands.

Mr. Transue—what a strange configuration, I thought. My grandfather and uncle are both math professors and go by "Doctor," while my brother is in computer programming with its informal styles of address. I've rarely heard any of the men in my family called "Mr. Transue."

We took him out for lunch with Arnold at a nearby restaurant. We chose a quiet table near the window. "The noise confuses him," Arnold explained. He ordered my father a rare hamburger. "He has a passion for almost raw burgers; this is the only place that satisfies him," he noted in a humorous undertone to Chris.

Chris grinned and his eyes met mine; I, too, like my burgers undercooked. Maybe it's genetic.

Arnold and Chris sat on one side of the table while I sat with my father on the other, trying to help him eat his hamburger. The tomato and lettuce slipped out the back of the bun, coated in mustard and ketchup, dripping with grease. His hands became covered in bits of ground beef and bun and condiments. I poured ketchup for his fries after he struggled with the bottle, wiped his fingers carefully after he finished, dipped my napkin in water to wash the ketchup off his face.

As we were leaving the restaurant I took my father's hand. Mine were cold from stress and the crispness of the day. My father peered down at my white fingers.

"Your . . ." He couldn't come up with the word, so he skipped it. "Very cold." He turned to Chris. "Isn't that your job?"

Chris rubbed my fingers in the car. I realized this was the closest we would get to my father's blessing.

―――――――

"We should have a picture of the two of you together," Chris said as we were getting ready to go. "To send to your grandparents."

Obediently, I wheeled my father in front of a pretty flowering plant, and knelt at his side while Chris fiddled with the camera. My father looked confused for a moment, then cocked his head in sudden understanding. "You want to take my picture," he said. "You want a picture of the crazy person."

Posing for the camera, he shook his hands and twisted his face into his best imitation of a zombie. I winced, clenching my teeth with the effort of fighting back tears. The shutter clicked. I would be surprised later at how well the photograph turned out, my father's face asymmetric but not deformed, mine pained but not despairing. There was a visible connection between us in the picture that I did not feel in person, a tenderness, a peace. I would study it, wondering what Chris saw, and how this scene would have appeared to a stranger.

My grandmother put the photograph on her refrigerator. If you didn't look closely, it looked like just a happy father-daughter snapshot.

When I visited soon after planting my garden, Arnold was out of town. My father had gotten harder and harder to communicate with; fewer fragments of reality made it into his consciousness, and what came back out was less and less predictable. I realized I wasn't sure I could handle him by myself in a restaurant, particularly if he got upset or confused. I stopped on the way to the nursing home to buy a picnic for us instead. In the store, I filled my cart with every wonderful thing I could lay my hands on, as if this luxury could atone for every other guilt and sorrow. Cherries, out of season and expensive but irresistible in their red roundness, reminding me poignantly of that long-ago afternoon on the hospital lawn just after his surgery. Little blushing apricots, huge ripe peaches. Fresh-baked sourdough bread.

The soft, smelly cheeses that he used to love. I couldn't choose between the homemade limeade and freshly squeezed orange juice so I bought both, tossing them into the cart with an abandon beyond hope or reason. From the store's gourmet bakery, I added a tiny rich raspberry-chocolate torte, a pear and almond tart, and a large flat ginger cookie. I tossed in a mound of napkins and a few plastic forks and knives, and was ready to go at last.

The woman in line behind me studied my cart enviously, gave me a thoughtful look.

"Picnic?"

I nodded. I imagined that she thought I was planning a romantic tryst; I wondered what she would say if she knew the truth.

I pulled up to the low yellow building. Arbor House had changed its name to Windchime; maybe the former had not been adequately upbeat. I envisioned an ongoing progression of names—Whispering Reeds, Babbling Brook—evocations of pleasant sights and sounds notably devoid of language.

I led my father outside, and settled him into the car. He accepted my guidance passively. We drove to a park and settled at a table. I made attempts at conversation: "How are you?" "I missed you." He didn't answer or seem to understand, but I tried to keep talking anyway. I realized, to my pained surprise, how little I could think of to say.

After not very long I lapsed into silence. I smiled and held his hand, rubbed his shoulders, hoping that this would somehow be enough. That though we were robbed of the possibility of more complex communication, something would get through. I fed him, and he ate happily.

As we pulled back up in front of Windchime, I saw Jeff, a graduate student who was house-sitting for Arnold and who was also doing some things for my father, sitting in his car in front of the building. He hopped out of the car at my approach.

"I didn't realize you were going to be gone so long," he said, a little scoldingly. "He has a doctor's appointment. Had a doctor's appointment. We're late." He looked at his watch, reprovingly.

"I—I didn't know," I stuttered.

"I would have told you, but I didn't realize you'd be away so long—"

"I didn't know it mattered," I said.

"We'd better go," he said.

We agreed that my father shouldn't go inside, that it would just be confusing and take extra time. Jeff went to sign him out of my custody and into his own.

My father was confused, trying to follow Jeff inside. "Stay here," I said, contrite an instant later at my commanding tone. "Please, Daddy, just stay here."

"I have to go to the bathroom," my father said.

I was torn between distress at this further complication—I had already made them late, and now they would be later; he would have to go inside and use the bathroom and come back out again, who knew how long it would all take—and relief that this didn't happen earlier. I hadn't had a plan in mind for bathrooms. Could he go alone? What if he needed help? My mind veered away from the possibilities.

I led him inside, meekly accepted Jeff's frown of disapproval at our appearance. "He needed to go to the bathroom," I explained, and one of the staff led him off.

We watched their slow progress down the hallway.

"This will make an awfully long day for him," Jeff worried aloud, his voice half-concerned, half-chiding. "To have a long trip out and then a doctor's visit . . ." He shook his head.

"I'm sorry," I repeated helplessly. "If I had known—"

He sighed. "I just hope he doesn't get upset when we're there. He gets confused so easily when he's tired—"

"We were pretty quiet," I said. "I mean, we spent a lot of time sitting down—"

He looked up. "What did you do?"

"We went to the park, had a picnic."

"I worry about him getting dehydrated on hot days like this," he said.

I told him that I'd brought water, and limeade, and juice, and encouraged him to drink.

"Limeade was a good idea," he conceded, grudgingly.

I was suddenly stuck at how odd this conversation was, that I, the physician daughter, was being scolded by the linguistics graduate student over my father's hydration status. You can chide me for being a bad daughter if you like, I wanted to say, but I do know about fluids and electrolytes.

My father was bewildered at going back outside, at being expected to get back into the car with Jeff.

"What's going on?" he demanded, staring from one to the other of us.

"You have to go to the doctor," Jeff shouted.

"What?"

"The *doctor!*"

"I don't need any dinner," he said plaintively. "I just ate."

"No, not dinner, the doctor."

My father shook his head in incomprehension.

Sometimes he could understand printed words better than spoken ones. Jeff pulled a notebook out of the car, and printed in large letters: DOCTOR.

"Why are you going to the doctor?" my father asked.

"Not me. You," Jeff said.

"What?"

"You," I shouted, in turn.

He turned away from both of us.

Working in concord now, we abandoned explanations and started trying to get him into the car. With a series of ludicrously exaggerated hand gestures we directed him to the front seat.

"Okay, okay," he said. With one of us on either arm, he eased into position to get into the car. But at the last moment, he twisted too far, landing in the seat facing almost backwards.

"Not like that, Daddy—"

He was staring into the backseat now, studying it with interest. I climbed in on the driver's side, and Jeff and I together tried to shift him around. We got him turned partway, facing out the passenger door, when suddenly he flopped back, across the center console, dropping his head into the driver's seat. I jerked back so he didn't hit me.

He lay there, staring at the ceiling of the car. "What do we do now?" he inquired, mournfully.

The question, so apt yet so inscrutable, lifted us from the tragic into the absurd. Jeff and I, simultaneously, burst out laughing.

When we were able to regain composure we lifted him back up, shifted him around, and settled him face-forward into the seat. He didn't look quite comfortable, but this would do.

I fastened his seatbelt and leaned to kiss his forehead.

"I need to go now," I said. "You go to the doctor. I have to go home to Seattle, but I'll come back."

He smiled the smile he's always used when he doesn't understand, sweet and a little wistful. His appointment to have the teeth out was coming up soon, and I still wondered how it would affect his smile.

"I love you," I said, my voice cracking on the words. I had promised myself I wouldn't cry in his presence, but I couldn't help it.

He reached up to my face, dipped his fingers into my tears. He studied me wonderingly.

"Oh," he said. "Oh." He frowned with a gentle, puzzled concern that seemed to contain no understanding, no knowledge of who I was or why I would be sad. His voice was at once familiar, a voice I knew from earliest childhood—that "oh," murmured as he cradled me to sleep, or picked me up when I fell on the beach—and ghostly.

I kissed him again, then watched them drive away.

15. BEING DOCTOR TRANSUE

Though I was ready to claim my title in defense of my ability to keep my father hydrated, I hadn't always been comfortable being called "Doctor."

I remember my first experiences with the title. Most of the people I worked with in medical school would refer to me as a medical student, but some used "student doctor," which was alarming, and a few went straight to "Doctor Transue," which made me squirm and want to wriggle away. "Doctor" implied I knew something I didn't; worse, that I was something I wasn't. I didn't want to cheapen the title I was working toward by claiming it too soon.

In private, among medical student friends, the word was titillating. "Someday you'll call me up and say, 'Dr. Chan, this is Dr. Transue, and I have a patient to refer to you.'" It's hard to remember now, how distant the title seemed then. It wasn't just a dream, after all. We were already on the road to becoming physicians, but we couldn't see the end of the path. We were like children trying on our parents' clothes; it was okay to play in them, but unimaginable that they would fit someday.

The year I applied to Dartmouth Medical School the cover picture on their catalog was of the graduation ceremony, a green-on-green stole—the green velvet of medicine and the green satin of Dartmouth— being draped over a young woman's neck. I wanted that. I wanted to be that young woman. Four years later, as my mentor slipped the stole over my academic garb, I had one of those rare flashes of triumph: "Look, I've done what I set out to do!"

I drove from New Hampshire to Seattle in a moving truck, followed by two nonmedical friends in a car. We communicated by CB, and I chose "Doc" as my handle. It's embarrassingly pompous and silly in retrospect; but I had only a week to get comfortable with the title before the rigors of internship began. Vermont, New York, Pennsylvania, Ohio: "Doc here," "Doc in," 'Doc out." I was a doctor. By the time we crossed the Mississippi, it started to feel real.

The honeymoon was short-lived. An intern quickly learns that "Doctor" does not mean, "someone respected for her hard work and accomplishments," but rather, "someone who can be constantly paged with questions, often trivial questions, and often in the middle of the night." Any romantic illusions I had about my title were quickly squelched by the endless repetition of phone calls. "Yes, this is Dr. Transue, answering a page. Okay, let's give him Tylenol, six-fifty, every four to six hours as needed. That's Dr. Transue. T-R-A-N-S-U-E. No, T as in Thomas, R-A-N-S as in Susan, U-E. Thanks." Who knew I would be so tormented by this title I fought so long to earn?

Slowly, though, my sense of identity as a physician began to grow. It happened almost imperceptibly, and often it took a glance through someone else's eyes to see myself in this new form. Midway through my internship, I was in the cafe at the Seattle Art Museum when a middle-aged man a few tables away clutched his chest and slid to the floor. I felt strangely helpless: In the hospital I would have known exactly what to do, but here I had no oxygen, no monitors, no medicines. The things I could do were simple: settle him on the floor, make sure he didn't hit his head, hold on to his pulse and listen to his breathing— happily, both were strong—and be ready to start CPR if either stopped. I pushed the stunned young waitress toward the phone and told her to call 911 and have them send an ambulance. I gathered some basic information on his history from his wife, and was ready to convey it quickly to the medics when they arrived.

I felt powerless at being unable to do more, and it was only after the medics bundled him up and left that I realized, by contrast, how powerful I felt inside the hospital. I hadn't considered before how good knowing what to do felt. I considered what a strange fierce joy awaited my colleagues on the other end of that ambulance ride, who would sweep him off for immediate treatment of the blocked coronary artery I could only guess he had. (I was right, and subsequently everything went fine, I later confirmed.) We go into medicine to help people, but it's easy to get caught up in the logistics and forget that we are indeed helping, and that it's a wonderful way to spend one's time.

After the ambulance pulled away I went into the museum gallery, as I'd originally planned. I felt strange, still flushed with adrenaline and still balancing the contradictory sensations of power and helplessness. As I was looking at a painting I heard someone nearby whisper, "Look! It's the doctor from the cafe!" Tears flooded unexpectedly to my eyes. I think it was my first moment of really feeling like a doctor.

At the beginning of my third year of residency I had another critical doctor-identity moment, also, oddly, outside the hospital. A college friend was visiting, one of those dear friends who nonetheless manages to slip in the occasional unexpectedly cutting comment. We were walking in downtown Seattle, repeating a discussion we had rather frequently in which he asked when I would become "a real doctor." I had already had my medical degree for several years, and was working eighty or more hours a week taking care of patients, so I found this conversation rather irritating. I was sick to death of the title he still used ironically—"People really call you, like, 'Doctor Transue?'" "Yes, hundreds of times a day." I explained that if by "real doctor" he meant having an MD, being able to write prescriptions, and having my own patients in the clinic and hospital, then I had already been doing that for two years. If he meant being able to hang up a shingle and practice independently, I could do that now if I wanted. If he meant being boarded in my specialty or being in private practice, that would be another year or two.

"I don't know," he said. "I just mean, being a real doctor."

"Can we talk about something else?"

"It's just—I mean, you're just you. Being a doctor, it just seems wrong."

At this moment, by pure coincidence, someone touched my shoulder. "Dr. Transue! I thought that was you!" It was one of my patients from clinic. I knew her well; she'd had some strange headaches the year before, and I diagnosed her with a brain aneurysm, which a neurosurgeon had successfully clipped.

After introducing her to my friend, I added, "How funny that you should appear just now. My friend here was just expressing disbelief that I could actually be a physician."

She spun on him with splendid, comic loyalty. "She saved my life," she said simply. It was arguable, of course; I hadn't done anything extraordinary. Still, it was a precious moment.

There were times over the years of feeling more or less like an imposter, interspersed with strange flashes of confidence. As an intern I guided a family through the process of withdrawing life support from their dying loved one. I answered their questions about what to expect, what we would do, what—as best we could guess—he might be experiencing. I stayed with them as we removed the breathing tube from his throat, and adjusted the medications we used to keep him comfortable as he was dying. I left them alone with him at the end, but hovered close by. His partner came out of the room to ask a question, and squeezed my hand tightly. "Thank you, for everything you've done."

"You're welcome," I said. Yet part of me was lost in wonderment that they should trust me to do this, entrust their loved one's dying to my care. What had I done, to deserve such faith?

Alongside the question of identity is that of self-presentation. In clinic, I introduce myself without a title: "I'm Emily Transue, it's nice to meet you." Of course, anyone seeing me in clinic already knows I'm a physician. I'm happy to be called "Emily" or "Dr. Transue," whichever any given person prefers to use. In the hospital, covering colleagues' patients, I introduce myself as "Dr. Transue" to avoid confusion. Then there's the question of coats. I wear a white coat in clinic, but I do it for practical reasons, not to make a statement. It holds all my essential doctor items: a prescription pad and a stethoscope, pens and business cards, and enough stray change to scrounge up chili in the cafeteria if I forget my wallet. Besides—a great bonus—someone else launders it for me.

At the hospital where I work, the people at the front desk recognize me if I have a stethoscope around my neck, even if I've forgotten my name tag. "Oh, hi, Dr. Transue, how's your day going?" Without the stethoscope, even with the tag, they sometimes don't recognize me and occasionally, if I've stopped to ask which room one of my patients has been admitted to, they'll offer me directions. With the stethoscope, I'm a familiar person in uniform; without it, I'm a stranger.

One afternoon, I went to see one of my oldest patients in the emergency room, where she was being evaluated for chest pain. I was without either stethoscope or coat, and she was in a little hospital gown, on a gurney. She reached out both arms to me for a hug, and I could see her nurse eyeing me, probably suspecting I was her granddaughter.

"I'm her primary care physician," I explained.

My patient jumped in to back me up. "She's my doctor. And isn't she just as cute as a button?"

It occurred to me that, with a few years' less experience under my belt, I would have been mortified by that description. As it was, it was just fine.

In my second year in practice, I had a botched dental filling and needed a root canal. I'm irrationally terrified of dentistry, so I sat in the endodontist's stylish office carefully talking myself down from panic. I filled out the forms, interested to notice that the endodontist, unlike my dentist, had a box for "Dr." along with "Mr.," "Ms.," and "Mrs." on the name line. I checked the "Dr." box. It made me feel better, as though I were pulling some of the poise and confidence of my professional identity into this personal situation. I couldn't accept the incongruity of marking "Doctor" and then wanting to run away or call my mother on my cell phone. I sat calmly and willed myself to feel better. I was alone in the room for a few minutes, until another patient filled out her own forms and took a seat.

"They made me give a photo ID," she commented. "What do they think, that I might be using someone else's insurance?"

This reminded me of a story. "Stranger things have happened."

She raised her eyebrows, so I went on. "A couple years ago a guy came in to the hospital with a cough and an X-ray that looked like it could be tuberculosis. They didn't bother testing for it because he'd just been in the week before and his tests had been negative. Turned out it was a different guy; a group of illegal immigrants were sharing the same name and social security number. He did have TB, and it was a mess. So, maybe photo IDs aren't such a bad idea."

"Are you a hospital nurse?" she asked.

"Actually I'm a doc." "Doc," my CB handle from that cross-country drive so many years ago, is now the word I use when I have to give a title but don't want to sound uppity about it. If her tone had been condescending I might have said, "I'm a physician," instead.

"Dr. Transue?" The endodontist's aide was standing at the door, holding my chart. I'd just written down the title on the form, but still it startled me to hear her use it. "Just this way."

One morning in the hospital, my patient's wife gave me a conspiratorial smile. "Did you have a good run this morning?"

"Excuse me?"

"Our nurse said he sees you running around Capitol Hill."

"Really?" I blushed unreasonably. "Yes. Yes, I do, and yes, it was a good run this morning. I never realized anyone was watching—" Even as I protested, I felt a warm flush of belonging. Belonging to my city, my neighborhood, my house, my running route . . . and yes, my patients, too. I was beginning to feel it, as they came back again over weeks and months and finally years. Many came in referred by others: "My mother-in-law just thinks you're terrific." "The girls at the office are all making appointments to see you. . . ." I knew better than to think too much of this; I'm personable, I'm a good listener, I don't have too long a waiting list. Those aren't such special things, and they're enough. Still: my patients. A strange warm feeling settled over me, a sense of belonging, of having a place. *This is my practice. I am Dr. Transue.*

16. MUSINGS ON DEATH FROM A DAY IN JANUARY

Medical diagnoses often seem to cluster; you may go years without seeing a patient with a particular problem, then see several in a few weeks or days. Statistically, this is the nature of chaotic events, but it can feel strange, as though an invisible hand were rearranging your schedule to bring a number of people with a certain problem to your attention. One morning, I saw five people complaining of leg swelling, leading the medical student who was with me to wonder aloud if we were witnessing the cusp of an unidentified epidemic. The next time she came, everyone had heartburn instead. Sometimes the cluster is not a symptom but a circumstance: all of the day's patients seem to be getting married, or getting divorced. Much of this, of course, is also the observer's bias; once you're attuned to a particular issue, you can begin to see it everywhere.

Perhaps it was I, as much as my patients, who was thinking about death on this particular morning. My father's partner had made the decision to enroll him in hospice care. My grandmother was in the hospital again with intestinal bleeding. Realistically, when your profession revolves around health and sickness, questions of life and death are never more than a small reach away. Still, as the day went on, it seemed that everyone I talked to touched on the idea of death in one way or another.

My first visit of the morning was to the hospital, where Adam

Farmer was waiting to have his colon taken out for intractable ulcerative colitis. "Hamburger" was the word the GI doctor used to describe his colon tissue in the sigmoidoscopy report. Neither Adam nor I missed the irony that hamburger was one of Adam's favorite foods. He was a single dad to a young daughter. She was staying with his sister while he was in the hospital, and he spent hours on the phone with her every day.

The nurse was talking to him as I walked in. "No, the social worker doesn't have a form for wills. Just durable power of attorney. You know, medical things." Are wills not medical, I wondered? Have we declared death outside our purview? "You'll have to get a lawyer," the nurse said.

"I don't need a lawyer," he answered. "I just need a notebook. If someone could go down to the gift shop and get me some kind of a notebook—It won't be hard. There are just a few things I have to write down."

Walking in on this, I was tempted to tease, to try to coax him out of his seriousness. He was young, and healthy overall; he was going to come through the surgery just fine.

But I thought better of the dismissive approach. "You're not going to die," I said. "But if you like, I can go down and get you a notebook."

He nodded.

Later in the morning, a son recounted to me his mother's final words. "Get out," she'd said. "You're breathing my air."

After him, I saw woman in her seventies who volunteered with pediatric AIDS patients at the hospital. She came in because she was having trouble sleeping.

"Is there anything going on that's making you anxious or worried?" I asked.

"The work is fine, the work is wonderful—" She always reassured me about this; I think she was afraid that I would say something that would make the people at the hospital think the role was too hard for her. Her last visit had been for back pain. "I think, maybe, that it might have gotten just a little worse from carrying the kids," she'd said. "But just a little. Don't tell anyone." She was plump and rosy-cheeked and terribly polite.

"Are there other things, besides the work?"

"Well, my sister—my sister's dying. I told you that before. Her heart's giving out, she can't breathe. . . . The doctors say it won't be long."

"I'm so sorry."

"It's okay. I know—I know things like this happen. It's part of life; at my age, you learn to understand."

I nodded.

"That's not what gets to me. What gets me is her husband. He doesn't care. He treats her like she's just there to take care of him, the way she always has.

"He's got Alzheimer's. He doesn't understand. I know, he doesn't know, he can't.

"But he's just so happy. He's just dumb and happy, and still expecting her to wait on him, and he's just . . . he's a shit." She said the word emphatically. "He always has been. He ought to suffer. I can't stand to see him so happy, when she's suffering, when he's the one who deserves to die, not her."

She stopped, and her eyes widened in horror at what had just escaped her mouth. But she lifted her jaw, resolutely, and I could see her deciding not to apologize.

"Can you give me something to help me sleep? When I've been up all night fuming, it's hard to keep my energy up at the hospital."

As I sat at my desk documenting her sleeping prescription, my medical assistant appeared in the doorway. "Hey, you know Willard?"

Did I know Willard. . . . Willard of the tree-trunk legs, weeping fluid and pus, Willard of the terrible shortness of breath and the intractable back pain. Worst of all, Willard of the three warring daughters.

Within a week of my first visit with Willard my medical assistant had logged thirty-two calls from his daughters, each denying everything that was said by the others, and each laying out her own set of demands for Willard's care. Willard himself sat, wide-eyed and blinking, agreeing with whichever one was in the room and otherwise not saying a word.

It was the hardest two weeks I had had in practice before he was admitted to a nursing home for temporary wound care. This particular nursing home had its own dedicated doctor, so we had a respite from the barrage of phone calls for a few weeks at least.

I was dreading what my medical assistant was surely about to say: his legs were better and he was coming back.

"He died," she said. "I saw his obituary in the paper yesterday."

Her eyes were on me, and my flip comment was silenced before it formed: *Thank God, those crazy women won't be coming back.*

"That's sad," I said.

She nodded. But she looked uncertain, and I realized I needed to admit the unspoken before she'd accept anything else.

"His family is a real pain, okay. But poor Willard."

"Yes." This time she could see I meant it.

After work I would find the paper and read his obituary. It started by listing his survivors, and I couldn't suppress a cringe. Then it talked about his purple heart for valor in the military, the wife he loved who died young in a boating accident. Then the business he founded and led, and the work he did for the international human rights movement. A Willard I never saw, and never dreamed existed.

It felt strangely better, to be able to mourn the man he really was.

Thinking about Willard and wondering what it had been like for him at the end, I remembered a recent careless conversation with a friend who doesn't work in medicine. "Medical people are callous about death, of course," he said. "You have to be. All this do-not-resuscitate stuff and this talk of 'good deaths . . .' I understand you need to think that way. But for someone who's actually dying—or for someone who loves them—of course they want to fight, to do everything they can. It's the only life they have."

What do you know about it? I wanted to retort, holding back out of politeness. How can you call me callous, when you have never wept with me at a bedside? Can you really think that there are not people who are ready to face death, that the decisions to stop fighting are a creation of the medical establishment, we who so often push things so much harder and longer than a peaceful soul in a troubled body might wish?

A fax had come out of the blue two days earlier, from one of the local hospice organizations, about Liz Williams, my patient with the metastatic gallbladder cancer. It was a request for an authorization for pain medication, back-dated by several weeks.

She had disappeared soon after her diagnosis was made. I had tried to reach her when she stopped coming for appointments, and finally concluded that she'd moved out of town; she'd talked about doing that, immediately following and even prior to her diagnosis. There was no answer or voice mail on her phone; none of the other doctors who had been caring for her had seen her, either. Moved away, then, I guessed—until the fax came. She was still in Seattle, and she was on hospice. I signed the papers; there was no need to delay her care while I figured out what was going on. "Get somebody from hospice on the phone," I told my medical assistant. "Somebody who can tell me what's going on with Liz. Where she is, how she is. . . . She must be seeing some other doc outside our system, and they sent me this by mistake. I'm happy to do the paperwork, but I want to know what's going on."

My medical assistant called, and the hospice person was supposed to call us back, but he didn't, and I . . . I forgot. Caught up in other things.

Now, two days later, there was another fax. This time I called myself, instead of delegating it. "I need to talk to someone who knows something about Liz Williams."

I sat for five minutes on hold, while a new patient waited for me in my examining room. I was transferred from desk to desk: nobody could find anyone who knew her, someone who did was on vacation, someone else was out on a home visit.

Finally the breakthrough came. "I found the social worker," said the voice on the phone. "She wants you to know she's not a nurse, and she doesn't know all the medical stuff. But she knows . . . she can tell you what . . ." She let slip the fatal tense. "What happened."

A moment later, a new voice on the phone. "This is Tina." Goodness, she sounded so young.

"Hi. This is Dr. Transue. Can you tell me about what happened with Liz?"

Tina's voice faltered. "I . . . well, she . . . well, it was hard at the end. She was doing really well, and then—suddenly she got really jaundiced, and confused. They were going to do some kind of scan—I don't really know that part—and she came in, and she was too agitated and confused to even do the test. And then—she didn't have a DNR on file. She hadn't signed the papers. I'd talked to her, I'd tried, but—she just wasn't ready.

"So they—they had to code her. It was hard. It wasn't a good end. She had a quick decline but it was rocky at the end."

The young voice on the line needed comfort that I didn't know how to give. "Thank you," I said. "Thank you for telling me. It means a lot to me to know."

The call had made me late for the new patient, who was in for a physical. I introduced myself and apologized for keeping her waiting. "It's fine," she said. Then she swallowed hard, and her eyes filled with tears.

Sometimes I think I have the effect of making people cry. People who seem fine when I walk in the door can be weeping ten seconds later, when I've barely said a word. All I had said was, "I'm sorry for keeping you waiting," and suddenly she was sobbing.

"I'm sorry—" she said, as I handed her a tissue. "It's dumb."

"No," I said. "Of course, it's not."

"It is, though. It's—it's my cat. My cat died." She sniffed. "I know that's dumb. But he was special. He used to leap into my arms when I walked in the door, and follow me from room to room like a dog. He would work his way under the covers when I was asleep, and when I played the piano he would sit beside me and reach out to touch a key with his paw sometimes. He was special."

"I understand," I said.

She dabbed at her eyes. "I'm sorry." She shook her head. "You deal with all these important things all day, and here I'm melting down on you about my cat. It's stupid."

"It's not," I said. "You love him. He's been a part of your life for years; he made you happy. He was part of your family. That's important."

I really meant it. Pets can be knit as tightly into people's worlds as human loved ones, and losing them is terrible. Still, I thought of Liz Williams, dying in a blaze of shocks and chest compressions, not ready, not at peace. An unimaginable horror. I tried to hold the woman's grief over her cat and the news of Liz's death in my mind at the same time: they were both real, but they didn't seem to fit inside my head together. I schooled myself to be present with the woman in front of me, to be with her in her sorrow. There would be time to grieve for Liz later.

17. INTERRUPTIONS

Staying focused on the person you're with is always a challenge. Putting everyone else, however sick and complicated, out of your mind is hard enough; on top of that, there is the constant stream of interruptions.

I believe that I have heard, in my years in practice, every cell phone ring known to humankind. From the softest twang to the loudest jangle, baroque to reggae, rap to ragtime—I've heard phones that seem to play whole movements of symphonies. Most people whose cell phones go off during their visit are a little embarrassed. Some are not, and there are always the few who answer the phone—it's rarely an emergency—chat for a bit about this and that, and finally say, "Hey, I'm at my doctor's, I have to go."

I don't really mind the phones ringing. My patients have jobs, have children and sick parents; they need to be reachable in emergencies. It can be frustrating, but it's not a big deal. There's the initial ring, the more insistent ring as the seconds pass, then the fussing through pockets and bags to find the phone. Often there's a second, different ring twenty seconds later indicating that the caller has left a message. It would be ideal if everyone could turn their phones off on the way in and check for messages after they leave, but I'm okay with a looser etiquette. It seems reasonable to hear the phone, check the incoming number, and either switch it off or do a five-second "I'm at the doctor's, is it an emergency? I'll call back, bye." This is not always how it plays out.

"Hello? Yes, it's me."

Pause.

"Really?"

An even longer pause.

"Really?"

"Oh my God, you've got to be kidding. And what did *you* say?"

"I can't believe it. What are you going to do?"

"That's crazy!"

"I really can't believe it! Well, anyway, I should probably get going. . . ."

On the few occasions when I've actually had to leave the room because of an ongoing cell phone conversation of no apparent significance, I almost didn't go back in. I entertained fantasies of leaving the patient in there until their cell phone batteries ran out, then hoping they would just drift away.

Sometimes it isn't actually my patient who's on the phone, but someone they brought with them. Guests in the room often seem to feel free to have prolonged chats on their cell phones, sometimes at a louder volume than the conversation I'm having with the patient. Apparently the cell reception in my exam rooms is not very good, so there's a need to yell.

"Are you having any chest pain?" I was asking a patient once, while her friend sat in the chair beside her.

"Well, I—"

The opening notes of Bach's *Cantata and Fugue* burst from the accompanying friend's breast pocket, at steadily escalating volume.

"Hello? Susan! I'm so glad you called!!"

"Well sometimes I have a little ache . . ." my patient managed to get in.

"I've been wanting to catch up forever!!"

"Where in your chest is—"

"So what have you been up to?"

Another time a woman's cell phone dialed 911, of its own accord, from her purse while she was in the office. Her grandson had programmed the phone with 911 on speed dial, and somehow the button was pushed as her leg rested against her bag. The telephone made a noise and she reached in and hung it up, not knowing what had happened. The 911 dispatcher called back to identify the emergency, leading to great confusion all around. She was finally able to persuade him that, really, she was all right. She handed the phone to me, so that I could professionally attest to her good health.

Cell phones are the most common, but not the only, source of interruptions in the office. Children are another popular one. We don't encourage people to bring their kids to their visits. I like children, but since I only take care of adults my rooms aren't childproofed, and there's a safety issue—not to mention the difficulty of trying to focus on the patient's needs while an infant is wailing or a toddler is tumbling around the room trying to dislodge loose, possibly sharp objects. But I take care of many young mothers, and I understand that they can't always find child care. I had a young woman come in once complaining of fatigue and headaches, accompanied by four children all under the age of six. I had to pop a few aspirin myself and rest my head on the desk after they were gone.

Many of the children, of course, are delightful. One young parent parked a stroller in the corner of the room; I couldn't see the baby, but he was quiet so I assumed he was asleep. A few moments later a small clear voice came from the carriage.

"A," the little voice said thoughtfully.

I looked up in surprise, but when nothing followed, the mother and I continued our discussion.

"B. C."

He continued murmuring contentedly to himself, letters wafting up intermittently, until he got to G—he missed F—then started over.

I, of course, garner interruptions, too. I don't wear my pager during the day (my calls come in to my office instead, during business hours) but my staff will occasionally tap on the door to pull me out for a call from the hospital or emergency room, or an urgent question from a colleague. We try to keep these interruptions to a minimum, but they do happen. I have never quite understood, though, why I'll have no interruptions for days, and then several in the course of one patient visit. The first is fine. "I'm sorry, I'll be back in just a sec—"

The second is harder. "Again! I'm so sorry. This never happens. Do you have something to read? Really, I'll be right back."

But the third is terrible. "Okay, this is getting ridiculous. I feel like I should offer you a free drink, like the airlines. Do you need to make any calls on your cell phone?"

Some interruptions are more disruptive than others. Once my receptionist tapped on the exam room door. "It's Dr. Johnston from the ER on the phone . . ."

"I'm so sorry, I'll be right back," I told my patient.

"Emily, it's about your patient, Andrea Jefferson."

He paused, seeming to expect that I would know the whole story from this much information. The name didn't sound familiar, but I'm horrible with names. In the middle of my freshman year in college I was introducing my roommate to someone and suddenly couldn't come up with her name; the same failure to produce a name, or a face to go with one, still plagues me.

"I'm not immediately remembering who she is," I confessed to the ER physician.

"You know her, you see her all the time, you just saw her last week."

"Remind me, real quick . . ."

Holding my hand over the phone, I gesticulated wildly to my receptionist to get me the chart, *fast*, please.

"She came in having a seizure. I guess she's been doing a lot of that. She's had a history of a lot of bad drug reactions, so I tried to give her just a small dose of diazepam, but eventually we had to give her more. And we still couldn't get the seizure to stop, and then she stopped breathing, and we had to intubate her.

"I guess the original lesion was thought to be from a subarachnoid hemorrhage, or that's what I understand; you know a lot more about what's going on than I do," he said. "So, anyway, we'll scan her and get her up to the Intensive Care Unit, but you better try to get here as fast as possible. . . ."

I tried to suppress the sinking in my heart, still wracking my brain—who was this woman?

"Okay," I said. "I'll just cancel my afternoon and come on up . . ."

Finally, I whispered meekly, "Do you happen to know who she has for a neurologist?"

"Excuse me?"

"Who's her neurologist?"

There was a pause, and then he sputtered, "Well, it says on the record that *you're* her neurologist."

I wasn't sure how to answer, so I said the obvious thing we both knew. "I'm not a neurologist."

"No, no, Emily, you're—"

There was a startled pause, and then a moment of understanding.

"I'm really sorry, Emily," he said. "We weren't looking for you. We wanted Stephanie Tran, from Neurology."

"That makes much more sense," I offered.

"Yes. Yes. Just—I'm really sorry. Just forget it, okay?"

My receptionist, meantime, was frantically tapping at the computer trying to locate a number and a chart for Andrea Jefferson, which we didn't have. She looked up, slightly panicked, as I approached. "Could there be another spelling . . . ?"

"It's okay," I said. "We're not supposed to have it."

I closed my eyes and tried to pull back the name, face, and story of the man in my examining room.

Sometimes it's even harder. A nervous tap came once on the door.

"Yes?" I poked my head out.

"Dr. Newbury on the phone," my medical assistant said apologetically. "He asked to have you interrupted."

"I'll be back in just a sec," I told the woman I was seeing. "I'm sorry." I tried to school my expression, to keep my face neutral. The call wasn't about her; she didn't need to see my dismay.

She nodded.

Eric Newbury is our breast radiologist; he does the mammograms, the ultrasounds, and the needle biopsies. He sends notes in little gray folders when the news is good. I hadn't gotten many phone calls from him.

"Uh-oh," I said as I picked up the phone.

"Nobody likes to talk to me," he said. "I'm starting to get a complex."

"I had a friend once who was a chemotherapy nurse," I said. "She ran into a patient in the grocery store and the patient threw up. Pavlovian conditioning. Talk about a complex."

"Maybe I should call sometimes just to say hi."

"Maybe. But that isn't why you're calling now."

"No."

"Who is it?"

"Green," he said. "Kelly Green."

It took a moment for me to call up her face. Pretty, red hair, slightly plump. Anxious—anxious already, about her marriage, her kids, even before she came in a few days ago with the lump. And—young.

"Thirty-seven," Eric was saying. "You saw her Wednesday, we did the studies and the fine needle aspiration yesterday. Three centimeters high grade ductal carcinoma."

"Damn," I whispered. Then, recollecting myself, "Sorry . . ."

"Don't be; entirely appropriate."

"I'll talk to her. Thank you for calling."

"Wish I hadn't had to, but you're welcome anyway."

I set aside the piece of paper; I'd call her a little later, when I had a break. I tried to refocus on the person waiting in my room, as if the world hadn't just shifted under me.

I walked back in. "Sorry about the interruption; where were we?"

———

Once I was interrupted silently, not by my staff but by a migraine aura. I've had half a dozen of these in my life, and this one began like the others, with a small sparkle in my peripheral vision that grew steadily into a fireworks display obscuring half my sight. I was seeing someone for a checkup; we were in the talking rather than the examining stage, and I was running late. I considered mentioning to the patient that half her face and body along with the left side of the room had been taken over by a whirling, jagged fireball, but I decided that she would probably find this unreassuring. If I excused myself for the duration of the aura I would then be even more late, with a headache descending besides. So I waited it out in silence. Happily, I could see again by the time I had to examine her.

Other times the interruptions come from something entirely external. The city cut down a tree outside the clinic once, and ran the branches through a wood chipper while I was seeing patients. We were in a windowless exam room, and the sound was so intense it was difficult to identify or localize. In a break in the noise, the woman I was seeing said seriously, "I don't want to have whatever procedure that person is having."

Another time I was interrupted by a seismic event. It was a beautiful February morning in my first year in practice, and I was waiting outside the exam room while a seventy-year-old got undressed for her physical. Her brother, who suffered from anxiety and panic attacks, was next on my schedule and was in the waiting room.

Suddenly the earth began to move. It trembled, wriggled, paused for a moment, then downright shook. I looked out the window and saw the small steeple fall from the neighboring church. I had never been in an earthquake, and it took me several seconds to figure out what was happening. "I've heard of this—wait, yes, this is an earthquake!" Then someone called out, "Get into the doorway!" and I heard the anxious man in the waiting room scream. It was a very long earthquake—later reports confirmed the shaking continued for forty-five seconds—and I had time to get into the doorway along with the anxious man, and to consider, bizarrely, the fortuitous fact that I had secured earthquake insurance for my house just a few weeks before.

At long last the movement stopped. The anxious man sank to the floor, still shaking although the ground was still. His sister in the exam room, who to my shame I had entirely forgotten, poked her head through the door.

"Can I get dressed? I don't think I really want a Pap today."

I looked down at my own trembling hands. "I think that would be just fine."

Every time I think I've seen or heard every possible interruption, something new comes along. There was the time I was examining a patient when a large book flew past me and slammed against the wall. Her husband had thrown it at a bee that had flown into the room, and was grinning ear to ear as its small yellow carcass fell to the floor. I startled easily for days after that.

My favorite, though, was Phil. I was about to do a Pap on a young woman, speculum poised in hand, when suddenly her backpack, which was on the floor at my feet, began to whine. Not an electronic whine but an unmistakable, organic whine. The pack was slightly unzipped and as I turned toward it a small, pointy furred head with enormous brown eyes poked out.

She glanced down. "Oh, that's Phil," she said. "I take him everywhere."

Phil stared at me with grave suspicion and I returned the look with similar mistrust. Finally he pulled his head back into the pack and the unmistakable slurping sound of a dog drinking water from a bowl began, followed by some satisfied crunching on kibbles. I looked from the backpack to the speculum, glanced up in appeal for sympathy to the distant heavens, and went ahead with her exam.

Later, I asked about birth control, which she wasn't using, and she said: "Oh, a baby would be fine. It couldn't be any more work than Phil."

Rarely am I entirely at a loss for words.

18. VALLEY OF THE SHADOW

The phone rang at eleven o'clock on a Thursday night in June. Work calls come in by pager rather than phone, and my friends know I go to sleep early, so they don't call late. I was in bed but awake; Chris was working in the next room. As the ringer sounded a second time I reached for the receiver, knowing that my father was dead.

Many people describe a sense of dread and finality as the phone rings, the foreknowledge of death. I was sure of what was coming as I picked up the line, but after all, I had known for weeks and even months that the call was going to come. Day and night, without being fully conscious of it, I was waiting for the phone to ring, for a tap on the exam room door at work ("Dr. Transue, I'm sorry to interrupt, it's a personal call"), for the answering machine to be blinking at home with too many messages. Now, in the dark of a summer night, it was time.

For years I had wondered what it would feel like when the call came. Even when I was child and my father first had cancer, I imagined in horror what it might be like if he died. In recent years, as his illness occupied an ever greater space in my mind, I wondered how I would feel when it was over. Had I lost so much of him already that I would have no grief left? Or would it all come back in a flash, each moment of loss from all these years, all those shards of sorrow suddenly fused together? Worst of all, might I be glad that after all these years of festering sadness, it was finally over?

Many emotions would come later, but in the first moment of hearing Arnold's voice—*Emily, it's Arnold. Jacques is dead. It was very peaceful*—what I felt was a strange sense of quiet. It was as though a great engine had been humming and grinding in the back of my mind for so many years I was no longer aware of hearing it, and now it had abruptly ceased. The silence wrapped around me, sifting and settling like snow. My next thought, as Arnold's words began to sink in, was that now I would need to call my grandmother.

There might be some uncertainty about a telephone call at eleven at night on the West coast, but at two in the morning on the East coast there was none. My grandparents' line rang for a long time. I could almost hear the telephone ringing on its little stand in the hallway beside their bedroom. I could hear her twitching out of sleep, reaching for the light, her bathrobe. Fumbling without glasses into the hall, knowing.

"Hello?"

"Grandmother, it's Emily."

Her voice cracked. "Is your father dead?"

"Yes."

She sobbed then, a howl of bereft motherhood that electrified the telephone line.

There is no cry like that of a mother who has lost her child. When I was working in the emergency room as a resident, there was a man who ran over his two-year-old daughter in his driveway. She was playing on the pavement and he couldn't see her as he backed up the truck. Her little body was crushed and crumpled, but the medics were still trying to revive her when they arrived in the ER, and we kept the effort going, the strangely different motions of child CPR in a place where we usually treated adults, actions I had learned about but never had to do before. We went on for half an hour, an hour, long past the time when there was any hope that she might live. We stopped only when there was no alternative to stopping.

I wasn't the one who told her family, who walked into the small peach-colored family conference room and spoke the words that ushered them out of the world they had lived in until today—a happy couple with a healthy toddler—and into the nightmarish place they would now inhabit, the baby dead, the father accidentally responsible. From down the hall I heard—we all heard—the mother scream. Her screams echoed through the front rooms where people were being examined for heart attacks and bleeding ulcers, and the trauma rooms with their gunshot wounds and car accident victims, and the back hallways where the drunks were waiting to be sober enough to leave. Everyone looked up, there in that place where nothing could surprise, because there was no sound like this sound, this otherworldly scream.

I thought of it now, listening to my grandmother wail. Even though my father was sixty-one and it was no one's fault and we had known so long that it was coming, it was the same scream. I felt I could have heard it without the telephone, from all those thousands of miles away. I wished that I could protect her, comfort her—and also that I could scream like this, let out my pain instead of holding in the stifled, strangled feeling in my chest.

Then she dropped the telephone and I could hear her moving into the bedroom to rouse my still-sleeping grandfather. "Bill, Bill, wake up—It's Emily on the phone. Jacques is dead. Jacques is dead."

On that repeated line I could feel it, finally. He was dead.

The other calls were not quite as hard. My brother, my uncle, my cousin. Finally I called my mother. They had divorced a quarter century ago, and hadn't communicated in years. Still—he was her children's father. Some ties aren't breakable.

She asked if I was okay, and finally I cried.

I went to work the day after my father died. My receptionist was horrified, misinterpreting this as an overriding dedication to work, rather than as my way of coping. What else was I going to do? Arnold was taking care of the arrangements, such as they were. My father's brain would go to the neurologists at Stanford, hopefully to add to medicine's understanding of post-radiation brain injury. His body would be cremated, and we would bury his ashes later in the summer, near the family house in Maine. He had hardly any possessions to disperse.

So I went to work, rather than stay at home alone with nothing to do and face the strange new silence. It was easier to be busy, to have the usual rhythms of my life around me. It helped to feel useful, the helplessness of those years of being unable to help my father suddenly brought into sharp relief.

Subtle variations of the obvious flitted through my head, each one oddly startling. *I have always been someone with a father, and now I am a person whose father died. For the rest of my life, my father will be dead.* My eyes filled with tears on and off, seemingly disconnected from my thoughts at any moment; I told at least one patient that my eyes were red because of allergies, an odd little lie. *What will fill the space that the sorrow and worry of my father's illness has occupied in my mind and heart all these years?* The silence was still there, a sense of time being suspended. Alone in my office between patients I felt delicate, bruised, not quite intact. In the exam room I did what I knew how to do. I listened to my patients' stories and did what I could to help them, and in return their grateful smiles quieted the ache inside me. I have often felt as though my patients healed me as much as I did them, but never so clearly as that day.

The next day—it was a Saturday—I pulled out the big box in the basement that holds all my personal letters. I went through piece by piece and pulled out all the letters from my father. It was not a thick pile when I was finished, and I read them through all, one by one. They were sweet, mostly short, and quotidian: accounts of working in the garden, little outings, commentary on the weather. If I was secretly hoping for something momentous—some gem of otherworldly truth, the key to all my unanswered questions about him, a coded message of fatherly wisdom sent from his younger, whole self to my older, grown one—I was disappointed. They were sweet, ordinary letters from a man to a child. But they were full of love, always. "You are a bright ray of sunshine in my heart," he wrote when I was eight (the letters, rare to begin with, became almost nonexistent when he got sick), "and you should always know the joy you spread around you." As the slim sheaf of papers fell from my hands I realized that this, after all, was all I needed. There would be no answers, and maybe there were no important questions. He loved me, I loved him. It was enough.

Now I was ready for tears, but they wouldn't come. Grief welled up inside me, and the emptiness of loss. The sun was setting, and the sky was pink. Chris was working at the hospital, but would be home soon.

I picked a faded, dusty book off the shelf. When I was seven, on a hot late afternoon in Toledo, Ohio, I remember getting to the page of Beth March's death in Louisa May Alcott's *Little Women*. It was before my father was sick, before anyone I knew had died. I cried and cried at the passage, which ends: "And those who loved her best smiled through their tears, and thanked God that Beth was well at last."

I reread the chapter now, and let the book fall on top of the pile of my father's letters, and wept. They were healing tears, the tears I couldn't cry in all those years of waiting, girding against the next little loss, the next little grief. Now it was over, and there was no longer a need to hold back. After all those years of half-grieving it was a relief, not that he was gone, but that I could mourn him fully. I cried, as the sun went down, and missed him, and was glad he was at peace.

19. THE MEDICAL HISTORY OF JULIA EVELYN (WILSON) HANSON

The practice of medicine is a good inoculation against self-pity. Each time you are tempted to indulge in feeling put upon—*why me, why did this have to happen to my father?*—you are quickly reminded that struggle is not an exception but a constant part of the human condition. Even more important, your patients remind you again and again of the ability of the human spirit to rise above adversity, to transcend grief and to triumph over the greatest challenges. I could hardly complain when I was constantly faced with people whose trials were far more difficult than mine.

Shortly after my father died I first met Julia Hanson. The greatest delight of my profession is the people you come to know, and Jaymes Hanson and his wife were among my very favorites. They had seen more than their share of difficulties in life, and had come through them together. After thirty odd years of marriage they still stared starry-eyed across my exam room at each other. I took care of her first, and then he asked to be my patient. My practice by this time had gotten very busy and I was limiting the number of new patients I saw, but I was glad to take him on. We always scheduled their appointments back to back, because they preferred to be in the room together. After one finished they'd switch places, a quick game of musical chairs between the seat and the examining table, and we'd start over with the other. They didn't ever like to be apart.

It wasn't long after I started seeing Jaymes that I came in to find a third person in the room with him and his wife. She was elderly, with clear, piercing eyes, sitting in a walker with a seat that doubled as a chair. As I walked in and blinked at her, surprised, she gave me the most thorough once-over I've ever experienced, studying me from head to toe. Then she stood up. "I'm Jaymes's mother," she said. "I'm not staying. But I'm looking for a new doc and I've heard good things about you. I wanted to see for myself. I think you'll do."

So it was that two weeks later I was presented with a typed document, in preparation for her visit. I sat down and began to read.

MEDICAL HISTORY OF
JULIA EVELYN (WILSON) HANSON

I was born on June 16, 1929, in Burley, Idaho, to Franz Joseph and Alma Phyllis (Hayden) Wilson. I underwent a tonsillectomy at an early age before starting school. The attending physician was Dr. Carruth.

I was married on July 23, 1944, to Jaymes Albert Hanson, a soldier in the Army Medical Corps. The following year, while he was overseas, I gave birth to a 5 lb 2 oz baby boy, on March 5, 1945. (Jaymes)

I gave birth to another son on April 10, 1953. (Alan)

I gave birth to a daughter on October 31, 1954. (Erica)

I gave birth to another daughter on August 23, 1956. Both girls weighed in at 7 lbs, 3 oz. (Betty Ann)

I gave birth to a stillborn daughter on October 2, 1958. She was deformed and had to be taken 6 weeks early at St. Stephen's Hospital in Spokane, WA. (Amy)

I gave birth to another daughter on January 19, 1961, at Greenacres Hospital in Lewiston, Idaho. (Annabel)

I gave birth to another daughter on February 4, 1963, at St. Peter's Hospital in Murray, Idaho, who because she was ill I could not care for. On the advice of my Doctor, I adopted her out. (?)

I gave birth to my last child, a daughter, on December 26, 1966, at St. Stephen's Hospital in Spokane, WA. (Stephanie)

I underwent a cholecystectomy on April 24, 1967, at St. Stephen's Hospital in Spokane, WA. My gallbladder had 6 gallstones in it.

I also have a history of ventricular tachycardia for which I have been hospitalized several times. The last time at Providence Hospital I had to be stabilized with electric paddles.

I have had several surgeries.

1. The cholecystectomy on April 24, 1967.
2. Modified radical mastectomy on May 9, 1991.
3. Knee replacement surgery.
4. Total hysterectomy.

I have Type 2 diabetes.
These are the medications I take.

1. Glipizide 5 mg. Twice daily for diabetes.
2. Metoprolol 25 mg. Two daily for heart.
3. Lovastatin 20 mg. Daily for cholesterol.
4. Baby Aspirin 81 mg. Daily for heart.

I have some other questions which I will ask about in person.
I will be happy to answer any and all questions needed.
Thank you.

Julia E. Hanson

There were pieces of the tale that made me smile: the careful accounting of the name of a long-dead surgeon, or the number of stones in a gallbladder. But my eyes were wet as I put down the document. I tried to imagine a life in which breast cancer would figure only in passing as item two in a catalog of surgeries. Or to think of the hardships sketched in those quick sentences with no hint of self-pity, the husband overseas at war for Jaymes's birth, the deformed child who "had to be taken early," lovingly listed with her name. The poignancy of the sick child who was given away on the doctor's advice, the simple but painful acknowledgment of not knowing what name she was given.

What a life to summarize in such plain language and simple strokes, I thought. I wondered what the questions would be that she had to ask me in person. I hoped I would be able to offer her something, to make the current chapter of this long journey better somehow. I felt honored to have the chance.

20. DOLLY PARTON

Most people look small in an ICU bed, but this one was minute, a tiny white-haired woman in her eighties, the size of a child. She seemed impossibly frail, with the tube down her throat and the ventilator taking steady breaths for her. The pneumonia had hit her suddenly and hard. Luckily her children found her in time, gasping on the bathroom floor. If I hadn't known her I'd have been convinced she wouldn't make it; there were bacteria in her blood, her oxygen levels were low even on the machine, and her kidneys were struggling. But I knew her, I knew she had great-grandchildren to look after, and gossip to collect, and jokes to tell. She wasn't going to give up easily.

Her children hovered close, a warm loving net around her.

"She's strong," I said. "I think she'll find a way to pull through."

I whispered her name, all six syllables of it, into her ear. She had a wonderful story about her name. Her father wanted a boy, and had a collection of short boy names picked out: Chip and Joe and Tim and Brad. When she emerged, disappointingly female, in a fit of pique he gave her the longest and most flowery name he could think of. "My name's always been bigger than I am," she would say, rolling her bright, huge brown eyes.

I whispered it now, again, and she opened her eyes and shivered. "You're going to be okay," I said, and she squeezed my hand. She tried to say something, but, of course, she couldn't speak around the breathing tube.

"Shh," I said. "You can't talk right now. Concentrate on getting better so we can get the tube out. Not being able to talk is probably the worst part, isn't it?"

She nodded and rolled her eyes. Being without speech is hard for everyone, but I couldn't imagine what it would be like for someone as wonderfully verbal as she was. She shrugged in frustration.

"You're strong," I repeated. "You can beat this."

She nodded.

It took almost three weeks, but finally the infection cleared and her lungs began to heal. We took the tube out and she was able to breathe on her own, though she was profoundly weak from prolonged inactivity and the lingering effects of the infection.

"She's a little like a wet noodle," her nurse warned as I headed toward her room on her first morning without the tube. It was an apt description. She raised her head just off the pillow as I came in, then lay impassively while I listened to her lungs and heart. Then she lifted her head again.

"Why are Dolly Parton's feet so small?" she whispered, her voice faint and hoarse, each syllable an effort. She knew I was a sucker for a joke.

"I don't know," I answered. "Why?"

But she was already falling asleep. "I don't remember," she murmured, the last word fading into a snore.

The next morning she was a little stronger; if she'd been a wet noodle, she was now al dente. It would take two weeks of rehab before she was strong enough to go home, but she would get there.

"Oh, doctor," she said, on her first visit back to clinic. "Thank you so much for saying I was strong. I didn't always believe it, but I think maybe you were right."

"Of course I was." I smiled. "By the way, I keep wondering—why *are* Dolly Parton's feet so small?"

She folded her small hands in her lap and giggled demurely. "They can't grow in the shade," she said.

WORDS

21. NORMAL

"Anything else on your mind today?"

It was my usual end-of-visit question, directed to a young woman who had come in for a sore throat. She paused. "Not really, but—"

"Yes?"

"My friends at work tell me this isn't normal."

She hopped gracefully off the bed, cocked her right foot outward, and dislocated her hip.

I stared for a moment in shock. "No," I said finally. "That's not normal. Please put it back."

She cheerfully acquiesced. "I can do the other one, too."

"Don't."

After a pause I regained my composure enough to have a conversation about lax joints and how she could protect herself from long-term cartilage damage. I was struck most by the way she introduced the subject, by that magical, hazy word I hear so often: *Normal.*

What is "normal"? Is "normal" what is average, common, expected? Or is it what is healthy, okay, free of harm or danger? Is it a statistical concept, or a form of judgment? My mathematical background leaps to provide an image: the normal curve, the bell curve. Is "normal" whatever fits within a standard deviation or two of the mean? On an intuitive level it makes sense to think that "normal" is what most of us are, and many medical tests are measured that way. But what is "normal" weight, if a huge proportion of Americans are obese? We define normal blood sugar not by averages but by what levels are associated with diabetic organ damage; with growing evidence we have steadily tweaked that number down, and the standards for cholesterol also. Here, "normal" is what's safe, what's least likely to get you in trouble.

At times I feel like a professional arbiter of normal. I'm asked questions about normalcy that range from the merely murky to the completely unanswerable. What's a normal amount of menstrual bleeding or vaginal discharge for a young woman? How much is it normal for a man's urinary stream to change as he gets older? How many times per week or day is it normal to have a bowel movement? Is it normal to feel dizzy when you haven't eaten for five or six hours? What are normal ups and downs in mood and what's depression, what's normal stress and what's clinical anxiety? How is it normal to feel when your cat dies, or your mother gets cancer, or you lose a pregnancy at seven months, or you find your husband in bed with another woman at a party in your own house?

When I first started in practice, these questions baffled me. My training had mostly dealt with situations that were clearly beyond the pale of normalcy. I knew better how to deal with someone who was suicidal than with someone who wasn't entirely sure whether she was depressed. I could treat diabetes, but I had had no formal training in nutrition; if I knew that varying the way one ate could affect one's mood or energy, it was purely from personal experience. I knew all the causes of bloody diarrhea, but very little about why stools are sometimes thick and straight and other times look like rabbit pellets.

How was I supposed to answer these questions? The solutions evolved from a mix of common sense ("If eating sweets at lunch makes you feel horrible, don't do it"), personal experience ("I've had a pain just like that, and yours will probably go away just as mine did"), and extrapolation from the things I was sure of ("Your chest pain doesn't have any of the characteristics of heart pain; it's probably coming from somewhere else in your chest. You had a cough recently; maybe you strained a chest wall muscle."). I made heavy use of two common-sense rules that had never been made quite explicit in medical training. One, if something hasn't changed in a long time, it probably isn't dangerous. Bad things get worse, they rarely stay the same. Two, if something makes you uncomfortable or unhappy or keeps you from doing things you want to do, it's worth changing—even if the same symptom wouldn't be medically important in someone it didn't bother.

I viewed all this, in my first few years in practice, as cheating. People were consulting me for my professional opinion, and I was giving them guesswork and common sense. Why come to me for advice a friend or mother could dispense, or knowledge that the person asking already had inside herself?

Over time I came to realize that, in fact, there could be as much value in the opinions I thought were fuzzy or intuitive as in those I thought of as scientific. Sometimes people really did need to be told by an outside, affirming voice, what they already knew: that the chest pain wasn't dangerous; that grief was normal, but planning suicide wasn't. That they needed to quit smoking, or drink less, or exercise more. That dislocating a hip at will wasn't a good idea.

Other times what I thought of as guesswork was a much subtler thing: judgment. I might not know precisely whether someone's chest pain was from a pulled muscle or a spasm in the esophagus or inflammation around the rib; I might be guessing when I put one of these theories forward. I did know that it wasn't caused by the heart, which after all was the real question. I might not know why some people have always had three stools a day and others one every three days, but I could say with confidence that both were under that magic umbrella: *normal*.

22. LUCKY

Some people, of course, are absolutely anything but normal. The first time I met Nick Palmer, he leaned across the table to speak to me in a confidential tone. I had not yet said a word.

"Before we get started," he said, "there are some things I want you to understand."

I nodded.

"You're never going to hear any complaints from me. That's not something I do. I'm a man who's not supposed to be alive and I don't forget it."

I was trying to frame a comment, a question, when he whipped a sheet out of the briefcase lying at his feet. "Do you know what this is?"

I looked at it. It was a graph, a black line that sharply dropped from a spot marked "100" at the beginning down to "5" at a spot marked "year 2," and continued down from there.

"That's the mortality curve for metastatic cancer of the esophagus. I—," he pointed to a spot on the right of the graph, where the line had intersected with the X-axis, "I'm out here. I had it fifteen years ago. Everyone's supposed to be dead fifteen years out. I've been living all this while on borrowed time, and I don't ever forget how lucky I am."

He was a spry, slender man, looking much younger than his seventy years. His enormous eyes seemed to fill most of his face; thick glasses contributed to this effect but did not wholly explain it.

Once I had examined his mortality curve he let me ask a few questions. Any other medical problems? "Seizures. Been on Dilantin for decades, hadn't had a seizure in years." Medications? "Nothing but the Dilantin." Any other history? "No." Nothing else in seventy years? "No."

How had they treated his cancer? I asked. "Surgery, then chemotherapy. Oh—that's another thing you need to know."

"What?"

"No more of that."

"Tell me what you mean."

"Next time round, I'm not doing any of that. No surgery, no chemo. There were times in all of that when I wished I had just died. A man knows what he can take. I can take dying. I haven't got another round of all that treatment in me."

I nodded.

"I've got papers, explaining all this," he added, whipping another file out of the briefcase. I wondered for a morbid moment what else he had in there. "Advance directives, durable power of attorney. All that. It's written down, but I wanted you to understand."

"I understand."

At the end of the visit he hopped up out of the chair and reached for my hand. "I think you'll do," he said.

About six months later, I was nearly at the end of a very trying day. There were people scheduled for colds who turned out to also have suicidal depression, routine follow-up patients showing up with acute chest pain. I was forty minutes behind, enough to make both my staff and my patients edgy, as I walked in to my third-to-last patient. "Sore throat," the schedule said, booked for ten minutes. Excellent, I thought; I can be done with this in five, and I'll be five minutes less behind.

He'd been sitting there awhile, and he glanced up only momentarily from his magazine as I walked in. An older gentleman, slim, familiar. My first thought was that I'd met him once and there was something interesting about him, but I couldn't remember what. I hadn't had time to even glance at his chart.

He sat on the exam table; a woman, presumably his wife, was in the chair in the corner. She gave him a particular look, loving and exasperated. "You must have this your own way, mustn't you?" her eyes seemed to say.

"I'm sorry I'm late," I said.

"No trouble." He finished his page, unhurriedly, then finally set aside his magazine.

"So," I said. "Tell me about your throat."

Usually, I should point out, I don't open conversations this way. Usually I say, "Tell me what brings you in," or "What can I help you with today?"—something open-ended, an invitation to conversation. But I was anxious to take care of things and move on.

"First," he said, and my heart sank—no, no "first" and whatever comes after, just the throat. Please, just this once? "I wanted to make sure you had all those papers."

"Papers?" I echoed weakly, defeated, lost. I had no idea what he was talking about—only that this wasn't going to take five minutes, or fifteen.

"Papers. All those papers we talked about last time. The durable power of attorney and all that. I need to make sure it's all in order . . ."

At that moment it all came rushing back. He was the man who had walked in and said, "I just want you to know from the start that you're never going to hear any complaints from me. I never forget how lucky I am."

"How long has your throat been bothering you?" I asked.

"About a month. But I want to go over all the—"

He waved his hand, which he had been holding discreetly over his neck, obscuring my sight. There was no need to ask if it was just sore or if he'd felt any swelling. I could see the lump from where I was standing.

"I don't want any chemo. And I don't want to be in pain."

"Am I going to get to feel your neck at some point?" I asked gently.

"Maybe." He twinkled an unexpected smile. "But first—" He gestured toward the woman in the corner, who was still wearing her look of tender exasperation.

"This is my wife," he said.

"Emily Transue," I said, extending a hand. "It's a pleasure to meet you."

"Janice Palmer," she said.

"I wanted you two to have met," he said.

He came in alone for the biopsy results. I'd gotten the call from the pathologist that afternoon: cancer. Probably a different kind than the first one; a late effect of his treatment the first time, rather than a recurrence. It looked aggressive, either way. He would not get fifteen years this time; not even fifteen months.

I was surprised that his wife wasn't with him, and raised my eyebrows. "Where's your other half?"

"She had to take the nephew to the airport. She wanted to come but I didn't want to reschedule."

"We could've—" I began.

"No, no," he said. "It's fine." He shrugged. "The first time round, it's a big deal. They feel like they have to be with you for all this. The second time it's kinda old hat, you can go alone."

This isn't how these conversations usually go. Not that you can really put a "usually" on the you-have-cancer talk, but still, if you could, this wouldn't be it. . . . With a deep breath, I took the plunge.

"So. Your biospy result shows the lump is cancer."

"I was kinda going with that assumption," he replied dryly.

"I'm sorry," I said. "I wish I could tell you something else."

He squinted his enormous eyes at me. "I feel worse for you than I do for me. It must be brutal telling people things like this."

I couldn't suppress a smile. "You know, I'd have to go with it being easier on my end."

"So, what now?"

"What now" was a consultation with an otolaryngologist and an oncologist. He didn't want anything aggressive, he repeated; didn't I remember that from the first time we talked?

"Just talk to them," I said. "Listen to what they've got to offer.

Maybe there's something not too bad—maybe some radiation, or a minor surgery—that would buy you some time or quality of life. It's worth at least looking into it."

"Okay," he said. "We can look into it. But I'm not making any promises."

A few weeks later he showed up on my schedule for a physical. A *physical?* He was sitting in a gown on the edge of the exam table when I walked in. He looked almost as confused as I felt.

"So you're here for . . . ?"

"Somehow I got scheduled for a physical," he said. "I don't know what that's about. Your medical assistant said it's 'a wellness check.' I liked that. Wellness." He chuckled softly, bowing his wizened head. "But anyway. I don't think I particularly need my prostate checked."

"No, I don't think so either. I think we can go ahead and skip your cholesterol, too." He was not going to die of clogged arteries.

"You think?" He looked surprised that I should be so easily convinced. "Good. We're on the same page then."

"Good. So no physical, but I'm glad you're here. I've been wanting to catch up."

"I'm glad to see you, too, because I do have one question."

"What's that?"

"Do I have to keep taking this damned Dilantin I've been on?"

"I'd forgotten about your Dilantin."

"I haven't had a seizure since 1982. I don't drive anymore anyway. What's the big deal even if I have one? It's just a seizure. Worst-case scenario I hit my head and die; for God's sake, I'm dying anyway."

"Do you mind taking it?"

"Sure I mind taking it! It's like having cotton in my head for forty years. You can't think straight on that stuff. It weighs you down."

"You can stop it," I said.

"Really?" He sounded like a child who'd been told he could have ice cream for dinner.

"Go ahead and stop it. Call me if you have trouble."

"You always tell me such great things," he said, his tone carrying not the slightest note of irony.

"Okay, now that that's settled," I said, "tell me what's been going on."

"You wouldn't believe what I've been through since I last saw you . . ."

"I've gotten a couple of notes from the specialists."

"Yeah, I thought you might have. That was one of the reasons I wanted to come in. I didn't want you to think I was going back on what I said. *What the hell's he doing*, you were probably wondering . . ."

"No, not at all. But let's hear about it."

"So I go see the people you told me to see. At first, it seems like everything's going fine. I say no surgery, and they say okay. Your little oncologist—nice girl—suggests radiation, thinks that might get me some good time. So I say fine. I have no objection to time. So they send me to the radiation oncology guy and he starts poking and prodding.

"And he says: 'Of course, we're going to have to take your tongue out.'"

"What?" I squeaked.

He raised his eyebrows and nodded. "Well, to get to the place where they need to radiate. Apparently it's not easy to get to.

"So I say, 'You mean, take it out temporarily . . . ?'

"He says, 'No no, take it *out*.'

"And I say, 'There must be some kind of misunderstanding, thanks for your help, I'm just going to go ahead and go.'

"So then he says, 'Okay, not your whole tongue, we could get by with just a chunk of your tongue, and your voicebox.'

"*My voicebox!*" His voice cracked on the word. "As if never speaking again would be a fate any better than death." He took a deep, steadying breath. "Jesus Christ. Where are people getting these ideas? I've been very clear with everybody. Like I was with you. Was I not clear?"

"You were very clear," I said.

"So, I'm thinking I'd better just go on down to Oregon. They've got laws down there, you know . . ." Oregon's assisted-suicide law comes up often enough in conversations with terminal patients that "going to Oregon" has assumed a second meaning. "And it's important that it all be legal. I've got my wife to think of, I can't have my estate tied up in probate—"

"Hold up, hold up, hold up—" I said, my mind spinning.

He didn't pause. "So how does it get you, something like this? Everyone keeps saying it's an ugly way to die but nobody says anything more than that."

He fell quiet for the first time in the interview, looking at me expectantly.

"Nick, I . . . that's . . . that's not a question anyone can really answer. I can give you some ideas, but nobody can tell you for sure."

"Tell me more or less, then."

"Well, it's in your neck. It can grow to where you can't swallow and you starve unless we feed you some other way. It can grow into the trachea and cut off breathing. It's not all that close to your carotid arteries, but in theory it could grow into one and you could bleed. Or it could make you susceptible to an infection that could kill you."

He didn't seem alarmed; he nodded calmly. " 'Most everybody seems to think I'll choke to death."

"But Nick, for any of those things—it's not like we just leave you to choke, or whatever it is. There are things we can do so you wouldn't suffer."

He shook his head. "They said they can't palliate it. That's what both those doctors said."

He pulled out of his briefcase (I recognized it as the same briefcase from which he had previously pulled the mortality curves and legal papers) a little pamphlet entitled, "Cancer dictionary," and showed me the definition for *palliate*. "To make less severe, without curing; reduce the pain or intensity of."

"They said that's not an option."

I thought quickly, trying to understand, racing through ideas and trying to edit my words at the same time.

"They may have meant—" What on earth could they have meant? "You have to remember specialists see things from a specialized point of view. The surgeon may have meant there was no surgical way to palliate it. But, . . . Well, to be blunt, there's always a way to palliate. There's always enough morphine to make you not feel what you don't want to be feeling. When the time comes, we'll use it."

"Really?"

"Really."

"Oh."

"When it comes time, one of the great tools we'll use is Hospice. They're the people who specialize in making everything comfortable and the way you want it to be at the end. They get involved when we think you've got about six months left. They don't hold you to it; they don't boot you out after six months for not being dead."

He grinned. There was a time in my career when I'd never have dreamed of saying something like that, but I've learned it can be the right thing. Levity in discussing death is not all bad.

"But yes, we can keep you comfortable. And we will."

"So I don't have to go running off to Oregon?"

"You don't have to go running off to Oregon. I promise. Not unless you want to see the Shakespeare festival."

He went back to see the radiation oncologist, and returned with a brighter report. "No cutting. But they said we should give radiation a shot anyway. It won't cure anything but they say it's easy and they think it'll slow things down." He shrugged. "I start tomorrow."

He was supposed to come back in a month, but he showed up a week early. "Thirty-six treatments," he explained. "I was supposed to get thirty-six. The first two weeks were fine, then all hell broke loose. I made it to seventeen; but no more. Every time I swallow it's like a red-hot poker ramming down my throat. You wouldn't believe."

"I'm so sorry—"

"Not your fault. But, fucking shit. I can't taste anything. Any God-damn thing I put in my mouth, it tastes like cardboard. Steak, bread, fruit, it's all like eating sand. The only thing I can eat is ice cream. Vanilla ice cream. Chocolate tastes funny. Then they tell me I can't have that."

"What?"

"They tell me I can't have ice cream. Milk products thicken your mucus, or something. Try soy, they say. So here I'm eating soy ice cream. Do you have any idea how vile—"

I interrupted him. "Eat the ice cream," I said.

"What?"

"Eat the ice cream. Did it make you feel worse?"

"No, it felt great. It was the only thing that made things—"

"Eat it."

"All right. Okay, that's better. Ice cream. As much as I want, whenever I want?"

"Yup."

"No soy."

"Drink whipping cream all day if you want," I said.

A few weeks later, his throat had healed. "I got back my taste. The taste of wine, and chocolate. The only thing I can't do is meat. My favorite little tender lamb chops—could just as well be cardboard. But I can live with that."

In another two weeks, he came back in for a visit with his wife. He felt good, back to normal. Too good, in fact, he explained confiden-tially.

"Doc, tell me; what's it all about?"

"I'm sorry?"

"What kind of pact have I made with God or the Devil here?"

"Ah, that."

"The math doesn't come out right. Everyone says, if we cut your tongue out and hack at your neck and God knows what all, then maybe you get two years. We don't know for sure. And everyone's all full of these gruesome you're-gonna-choke-to-death-on-your-own-spit stories. Then I get seventeen out of thirty-six treatments and here I am feeling fit as a fiddle. So what, they mangle you and you maybe get two years, and do pretty much nothing and you'll do fine for ten?"

"It hasn't been ten years, Nick," I pointed out gently. "It's been a month."

"I mean, what the hell is going on? It's terrible. I can't go on like this. What's next, they're gonna be telling me I'm dying of heart disease or a stroke and I'm gonna be ninety-five years old and still chugging along. . . . I feel better than I ever have! I think it's being off that medication. Since I'm off that Dilantin, I think more clearly. I'm more articulate.

"So people who haven't seen me in a while see me and say, 'You look terrific! You look better than you have in years. Why aren't you working, for God's sake? Why don't you do something useful with your life?' "

"Nick," Janice said, from her quiet perch in the back of the room. "I don't think—"

"And I think it's just being off that damned Dilantin."

I had to smile at all his swearing, and at the cheery tone in which he produced it.

"Nick—" I tried to clear my mind. "You made a deal with us, not with God or the Devil; with yourself, really. You put up with the radiation and how shitty it made you feel, and the benefit was shrinking this thing. It responded great. You felt worse than you or I had hoped, but it shrank down just like we wanted it to. That was the point."

He nodded.

"It's not gone. You know that. Sooner or later it's going to grow again. I can't tell you when, but it's going to come back—"

"Well, I sure hope it does. It's pretty uncomfortable living with this kind of thing." His tone was completely serious, and I willed myself not to laugh. "I've done it once already. Dodged the bullet. I don't know what I would do if I had to live with that again."

"You didn't dodge it this time. You delayed it a little. You're not going to live forever, if that's what's worrying you."

"I should hope not. A person isn't supposed to live forever. You don't want to be invincible. . . ." For almost the first time since I met him, he struggled for words. "It's strange, it's like a burden that you carry. When everyone's been telling you you're gonna die for so long and it never happens, you get in kind of a weird relationship with the world."

"I can see that," I said, although how could I truly conceive of what he was feeling? I can try to imagine getting a death sentence, but getting a second one fifteen years later? "But still . . . I wouldn't spend too much time agonizing over why you don't feel worse. You bought some time. Cherish it."

"Yeah, but—Goddamn. I've had everything a man could want. I've had time to see everybody, and say good-bye, and get everything taken care of. I've got all my affairs in order. But you give me too long, and my affairs are going to get back *out* of order." He leaned closer, dropped his voice to a whisper. "Dear Lord. My son's in some trouble about his taxes. I can't get involved in that."

He looked truly dismayed.

"Maybe I could write you a note," I suggested. "Please excuse Nick, even though he looks fine, he really is dying, and he can't get involved in any complicated family dynamics."

He giggled. "Maybe that'll work."

He was still chuckling as he walked out the door. Janice, who had sat shaking her head through the whole discussion, filed out behind him. I caught her arm.

"You okay?" I asked softly.

She nodded. I could see tears mounting in her eyes, but she didn't let them flow.

I sent the hospice folks out to see him not long after the new cancer was diagnosed. He said they were charming and wonderful but they didn't seem to know what to do with him. "They want to help me face death, but I've already pretty much done that."

"Well, you're not exactly a typical customer."

"So I'm not sick and I'm not struggling with my mortality, and I think I've got them a little befuddled. They keep offering me massages. I mean, a foot massage is nice, but . . ."

"Take it, then."

"But it feels like I'm wasting their time."

"Possibly, a little, for the moment. But that's okay. They'd much rather be involved early than too late to help."

He frowned.

"If having them around makes you feel like there are vultures waiting for you to get sick, call them off. But if it's nice to have them, let them keep coming. Take a massage or two now and they can do more later when you need it."

"I think they may like to come," he said. "I mean, you figure all day they deal with these people who are dying, and here's this chipper, fit old guy who's just waiting for a lump to grow, and we can chat and they can give me massages."

"Sounds fine."

"I'll think about it."

His wife called the next day to say he had decided he wanted them to keep coming. "I think the attention means more to him than he realizes. It's nice for an old man, to have some young folks fussing around him."

"Sounds good to me," I said.

It was the hospice nurse who called me when the lump reappeared. I thanked her, hung up the phone, and dialed his number. Janice answered.

"Are you doing okay?"

"I'm fine," she said. "Let me get Nick for you."

"Hey, doc," he said. "Sweet of you to call. Little bugger's popped up again."

"How're you feeling?"

"Not too bad yet. Hurts some. Each day's a little worse. Doc, we have to talk."

"Okay."

"I don't want to do this," he said. "I don't want to wait this out."

"Are you in pain?"

"No. They give me pills for that. But then I feel drugged. Neither way is good. Two bad options, and neither's getting better."

"We can adjust—"

"Doc," he interrupted me. "I know you mean well. But you're not listening. I don't want to wait this out."

There was a long pause.

"I've talked to the hospice people, and I understand their approach—comfort, and all that. Manage each symptom as it comes up. There's nothing wrong with that. But I don't want to do it."

"This doesn't seem like a good conversation for the phone," I said. "Why don't you come in?"

"Sure. I'll make an appointment. I've been doing some research—there's good books out there. Lots of useful information. And there's a local group called Assistance in Dying; I've got a call in to them and they'll be coming by. I've got some questions for you, though."

"Okay," I said. "I'll see what I can do."

"One more thing," he said. "While I'm waiting for the appointment. I can't sleep. I've tried that lorazepam, and the diazepam, and that expensive Ambien that everyone says is supposed to be so great. None of them does anything for me. I've read that this stuff called phenobarbital would be good to have around. I hear it's very good for sleeping."

I wrote him a prescription for phenobarbital. Enough to last a while.

He came in for his next appointment with his little black briefcase full to bursting. He pulled out a yellow legal notebook covered in scribbles.

"So when could you come out and give me my injection? I

understood that you might be able to give me an injection to get this taken care of—"

I suddenly felt sick to my stomach. How could I have given him such a completely wrong idea? "No, I cannot give you an injection!"

"But I thought you said drugs were okay, to make me comfortable."

"I could—we could—give you morphine, if you were having trouble breathing. Enough to make your breathing comfortable. Even if that meant you breathed slower and died faster than you would have—that's okay. I can't give it to you to make you stop breathing. Even if you want to."

"That seems silly. If living anyway at that point is suffering and you can stop the suffering in one way but not another."

I turned my palms out in a gesture of helplessness.

"So, no injection."

"Not like you're thinking, no."

"Not like I'm thinking, or not at all?"

"Nick—I respect your desire to control this, to control when and how it happens. But I can't help you control timing. I can help you control pain, when that times comes. I can't help you stop it from coming."

"Fine. No injection." I could hear him trying not to sound aggrieved. He drew a black line across a section of his notepad. "Okay, I guess that leaves pills."

He looked up. "The Assistance in Dying people who came out say I've got plenty of drugs to do the deed. But all the books are very insistent about the role of alcohol. Now, I'm not much of a drinker. But they seem to think it helps, chemically."

"Okay," I said, guardedly. He'd spooked me with his talk about injections.

"The problem is, they never tell you how much alcohol. I mean—am I supposed to down a fifth of whiskey? Two fifths? I haven't been a drinker in a long time, you know. I don't know how much I can hold."

He sighed peevishly. "I'd hate to just get snockered and forget what I was about. Wake up with a splitting headache instead of the Grand Exit."

I had to smile.

"Nick, I suspect if you were serious about this, a buzz wouldn't distract you."

"Okay, no. But, I'd hate to puke up all my drugs, then."

"How much would it take to get you buzzed without making you sick?"

"A shot, I guess. Maybe two." He gestured a measure with his hands.

"Well, then."

"Okay, I should take two shots?" He had his pen in hand.

I was still nervous. "If a person were theoretically trying to over-dose, they might want to drink enough to be drunk but not sick. I'm not saying you should do that. I think you shouldn't do that." I felt like I was playing Simon Says. *Simon Says the patient shouldn't kill himself.*

"You are instructing me not to do that. I understand." He made a notation on his sheet.

"So, when do you come, then? If you can't help. I mean, to con-firm I'm dead and all."

"Actually, I don't. The hospice folks can do that."

"So you go, what, to the morgue?"

"There's just a phone call, they call me to say what happened. The next day someone brings me a certificate to sign."

"You don't come out to see me—well, 'me,' however you want to put that—at all?"

"Nope."

He seemed offended.

"I can if you want . . ." I offered.

"No, it's okay."

He made another mark on his sheet, then looked up. "Why are you so scared about all this?" he asked suddenly.

"Mmm. I don't want to go to jail?"

"I understand that. I don't want you to go to jail, either. But the Assistance in Dying people aren't spooked, they seem to think it's fine. Why are you?"

"Their name isn't on the prescription bottle."

"Hell, girl, your name is on all my prescription bottles. Everything that comes in from hospice has your name on it and you probably don't even know what half of it is. I got some Bowel Kit the other day with your name on it—do you feel responsible for my Bowel Kit? What if I strangled myself with your enema tube?"

"Could you use your garden hose instead?"

"Okay. But—seriously. All games aside, it's not like you're encouraging me. This is my choice. I knew long before I met you that if it came to this, I'd make this choice. I'm of sound mind. I'm not depressed. I'm dead in a month anyway. You don't know for sure what I'm going to do; and if you did, you couldn't stop me. What're you supposed to do, call the cops and say you've got some dying guy you think might go and off himself?"

He fixed his round blue eyes on me sternly.

"I don't know. Maybe that is what I'm supposed to do."

He sighed. "You probably wish you'd never met me."

"No, Nick." I shook my head. "I would never wish that. I wish this whole thing were different. That you weren't sick, for one. And also that I could be more help. But I've been lucky to know you—I'd never trade that."

"Humoring an old man." He smiled, though, as he looked down at his notebook. "Well, I guess that's all my questions."

He hopped off the exam table. He always took the hard way: jumping off the side of the table, instead of sliding off the end where there's a step to stand on. It made him seem younger than he was.

"Keep in touch," I said, as he reached out to hug me.

"I will," he said. "But if I don't—take care. You're a good egg, doc. I'm glad I found you."

It was the hospice nurse who called, about three weeks later. I came out from seeing a patient and found a note on my desk. "Nick Palmer expired, 2:45 P.M."

I called Janice. "I'm so sorry—"

"He was ready," she said, her voice thick with fatigue and sadness. I realized that through all of this I'd never heard her voice any opinions, only constant support of whatever he wanted. I wondered how much she was holding inside, how hard it must have been to protect him from her grief. "He'd been ready for a couple of months. What can anyone say?"

I wanted to ask her how it had happened: what he'd done, or whether the cancer had taken him on its own. Faced, though, with the sorrow in her voice and the answering sadness rising in my heart, I realized that it didn't matter. He was dead. Neither the significance of his death nor the grief of those who mourned him hinged on the details of his last minutes. I would write on his death certificate that he had died of cancer, and it would be true.

"I'm sorry," I said again.

"It's okay," she said. "Thank you."

23. GRIEF

One of the strangest things about grief is how unpredictably it ebbs and flows. The triggers that strike most deeply can seem random and sometimes trivial. I have said this to many patients over the years, and I suppose I believed that knowing it would somehow let me bypass this aspect of my own experience—which, of course, it didn't.

For years through my father's illness, I cried at weddings. The very thought of a father walking a daughter down an aisle opened a floodgate into all the complicated sadness I had about my father. They were always distinguished and tender, those fathers in their suits and tuxes—their steps sure even when slow, their proferred arms strong, and their eyes aglow with pride. Father and daughter walking straight, each supporting the other, youth and maturity in a mutual embrace of love and protection. It was everything my father and I weren't, and I was haunted through the weddings of innocent friends by the image of my father with me in an imaginary church, with his twisted, demented smile, stumbling or flailing in his wheelchair, perhaps peering at me in uncertain identification. I cried for the imperfection of the relationship we'd had, for the amount I missed it anyway, for being deprived of the chance to make it better. I cried for the kind, tender father I remembered from my childhood and for the sad distance of those memories.

No amount of reason played any part in this. I wasn't planning a wedding. My father would have been much too sick to travel to a ceremony if I were having one. I had never really liked the idea of "giving away," with its implications of father passing ownership to husband; even if I'd wanted someone to walk me down an aisle, my stepfather, who in many ways played a larger role in my life than my father did, would have been happy to do the honors, as would my mother, who did the lion's share of raising me. I couldn't even cite a long-ago dream to explain my preoccupation; I had not had girlhood fantasies about standing in a poufy dress on my father's arm. None of it made sense, but somehow the walk down the aisle resonated into some deep inner chamber of my grief.

There were other things that made me cry, both before and after his death. Roses, because he always had particularly loved them. The summer after he died I found myself sobbing on a visit to the Portland Rose Garden, because he would have been so happy wandering in the maze of petals. A particularly good concert, or a dive from a canoe into a cold lake on a sunny day, could make me think of my father and be sad, knowing he would never feel that kind of joy again. On the other hand, the California poppies in my garden brought smiles, not tears. I couldn't put my finger on the difference.

Other sources of sorrow were more bizarre. It pained me to glance at the little Betty Crocker point squares on boxes of cereal and other foods. My father began collecting these when I was very young, carefully cutting the squares off the boxes and putting them into neat piles, telling me what wonderful things you could get if you collected enough points. I don't know that he ever actually sent any in. Eventually he gave the collection to me. He rarely sent me letters but when he did, a little pile of cereal box squares would invariably fall out. I piled them up loyally for years, never sent away for the book that explained how to redeem them, and finally threw them away, with a sense of crippling guilt. The optimism of his interest (wonderful things could happen from cereal boxes!), the touching though odd consistency of the gesture (all those years clipping cereal boxes, for me), the failure, first his and then mine, to follow through on it, and finally my own betrayal of his faithfulness and our unspoken keep-the-cereal-box-squares pact—all these were painful and bewildering. Trivial as the box-tops might have been, it is that combination of the touching and the pathetic that characterizes most precisely my feelings about my father.

All this happened before he developed the dementia. Later, the same drive morphed into an obsession with the sweepstakes ads that came to him in the mail. My father, to the end, was convinced that he had already won a million dollars. During my last visit to him, most of what I could understand of his conversation was worrying over his difficulties in finding the proper channels to claim his prize.

Some of the triggers for grief about my father were obvious. Throughout his illness I had a painful aversion to nursing homes, in general, and to dementia wards in particular. One excellent Seattle nursing home where I frequently saw patients had a wing called, with the Orwellian euphemism typical of such places, the Sheltered Freedom Unit. Like Windchime, my father's nursing home, Sheltered Freedom had a simple set of printed instructions explaining how to open its locked door, a way to let the cognitively intact come and go while those who couldn't decode the instructions were kept inside. I took care of a patient there, an older man with Alzheimer's (there was nobody on the ward as young as my father). My aversion to entering that hallway felt physical, magnetic, as if an invisible force were pushing me back when I tried to enter. I hated the faint odors of illness, which no amount of cleaning could eliminate, and the vacant faces of the residents, peppering the hallway in their wheelchairs like autumn leaves tossed and scattered by the wind. Each time I finished my visit I jabbed at the keypad with the exit code and slipped through the door just as it began to open, fleeing as though from a burning building. Even on the telephone, as a bland recorded voice circled through a directory—*Press two for Sheltered Freedom*—I felt myself recoil.

Along my way from home to work there is an old, grand Grecian mansion, a wedding cake of Corinthian columns and bannistered balconies. The year I started practice it was being renovated as a nursing home specializing in dementia care. I watched as they installed reinforced high railings on the balconies, and a tasteful but sturdy outer gate with the inevitable coded keypad. There were a series of signs: COMING SOON! NOW OPEN! Looking at the mansion and feeling guilty—that my father needed to be in an institution at all, that he wasn't here, that I wasn't nearer to him, that I didn't visit more often—became a part of my morning drive to work. Long ago, when my parents were first divorced, my brother and I used to drive with him from our house in Toledo, Ohio, to his in Columbus every other weekend. That drive was punctuated every half hour by landmarks: the parabolic tower of the nuclear power plant, the red-and-white checkered sugar mill, the clustered exits of small Ohio towns. On a smaller scale I checked off the landmarks of my drive to work: the stop sign, the house with the particularly pretty garden, the dementia home. Every morning the guilt hit as I turned that corner, the rest of my drive preoccupied with self-recrimination.

While my father was ill I dreaded Father's Day. All the media images were of doting dads, tender and wise, unerringly supportive, unfailingly practical; their children were faithful and adoring. Did the makers of the ads consider that not every father showed up with lumber and a tool box whenever something needed fixing? Or that sitting on the porch pouring out your heart to Dad and gathering his loving wisdom on the challenges of your adult life might not be a universal reality? "You've always been there for me," gushed the daughters in the Father's Day ads. "And I would do anything to give a little back." I gritted my teeth and averted my eyes from the media messages each June.

I don't mean to be melodramatic. I am stripped by my profession of the luxury of believing that any of this experience is novel, or even particularly rare. The human body is a fabulous, wondrous, yet fundamentally vulnerable thing. Every imaginable horror can befall it. We're not inured to this, as doctors, but we're less surprised by it than people who have seen less. We're deprived of the comfort of outrage, of the belief that illness offends some principle of order in the universe. My father's story strikes me simultaneously as unbearable and as perfectly ordinary. So my father had cancer. He survived and then he had a slow decline and died. It was terrible for him and everyone who loved him, including me. Still, things like this happen all the time. Worse things happen. Children die of cancer and teenagers kill themselves. People live in terrible pain and suffer immeasurably from human cruelty—my father had to bear neither of these. He lived many years after an illness that might have killed him. As for our relationship, maybe it wasn't the daughter-dad greeting-card fantasy, but then, how many people have that? He was kind, he was loving, he was not as present as some fathers but certainly not absent. Many, many people do worse. I have nothing to complain about.

"It could be worse." Patients tell me this a dozen times a week, usually in reference to something truly horrific happening in their lives. As I point out to them, this isn't much comfort; horror is not lessened by the specter of even greater horror. If anything, watching tragedies greater than my father's play out time after time in my practice made me feel worse. I wanted to be fists to the wind, calling down bolts of lightning, furious at the world for what was happening to my father. The quiet voice of reason and experience—*this isn't an affront against the world, it's the way the world is. This is the way things happen*—only left me emptier and colder.

After my father died I stopped crying at weddings, or at least stopped crying private, selfish tears. The thought, "My father can't walk me down the aisle because he died," was somehow more bearable than "My father can't walk me down the aisle because he can't walk and doesn't know who I am." The NOW ACCEPTING RESIDENTS! sign on the dementia home on the way to work became just a sign, not a coded message of reproach; and although I still cringed at the keypad to the Sheltered Freedom Unit, it didn't color the rest of my day as darkly. Father's Day now struck me as a piece of marketing built on myths of varying degrees of truth, not as a thoughtless piece of cruelty to the flawed children of sick or absent fathers. Many painful recollections became less so, and over time, more joy sifted into my memory. I could plant and dig in my garden and feel my father's motions in my hands with happiness and pride. I began to remember unexpected things: the songs he sang to me when I was a little girl, his voice wavering softly on the low notes; the motions of his hands when he cut a grapefruit. Joyful memories that had been buried for years under sad ones began to reemerge.

I've always been uncomfortable with the word "closure," the implication that at some point the door is simply shut on grief. The momentous events of our lives, both joyous and painful, will always be part of who we are. We can grow from a terrible loss, even heal to a point where it no longer hurts, but it never goes away.

The surgical sense of closure may be a better one. The last stage of surgery is closing the wound, bringing the cut edges back together so that the body can begin to knit them into a scar. An infected wound can't be closed; it will fester and break open. My father's illness was this kind of wound, each new stage reopening the tentative fibrils trying to mend the stage before. I grieved when he first forgot my name, then he remembered it for a while, and I grieved all over again the next time he forgot. I was pained at the moments that reminded me of who he once was, because of the contrast to who he had become, and pained again by the moments that failed to remind me. It's impossible to heal from a loss that isn't yet complete.

So my father's death did bring, after all, a kind of closure. As a wound might be after surgery, it was intensely painful; but the pain was clearer, simpler, than it had been before. It was the beginning of being able to heal.

24. WORDS

For every word like "closure" that raises my hackles, there are others that I love. I collect words, not in a static sense like pennies in a jar, but the way nineteenth-century Europeans collected orchids, searching them out, gathering, and tending them. Like an orchidist I remember the stories of my prizes, where I got them, and from whom.

I collect them, first, for use with patients. A word like "spirits" (a gift from my medical school mentor) is so much gentler and less laden than the harsher and more clinical "mood." "How are your spirits?" I ask a dozen times a day. Sometimes I combine it with another favorite phrase, "holding up": "How are your spirits holding up under all this?" I am much more likely to get a significant answer to this question than to the flat, "Have you been feeling depressed?" question I was taught in medical school. Perhaps my very favorite word is "struggled": "How long have you been struggling with anxiety?" It's more active, more positive than "suffered," that sad old medical standby. "Struggle" has a nice little political edge: "How long did your mother struggle with the breast cancer?" Another favorite, "regularly": "Have you ever smoked regularly?" I don't need to hear about that one night coughing your lungs out in your high school best friend's car.

I delight in new phrases I have cooked up. Over dinner one night a friend complained about the phrase, "trying to get pregnant." Intimations of failure, she said, and also an unfortunate evocation of the act of the effort. Over sushi we rejected the similarly burdened "hoping to get pregnant," and the overly vague "thinking of a pregnancy," and arrived finally at "wanting to be pregnant," which I have now been using with the delight of a child testing out a new toy.

Then there are those phrases I have not yet found. A good substitute wording for "Are you sexually active?" eludes me. The original has earned me blank looks from many patients, and from one, an interested gaze around the room, as if in search of a hidden something or someone, followed by an oddly unironic, "Not just at the moment. . . ."

I carefully cull out the weeds, the words I do not want to grow: "discomfort," "procedure," "neoplasm," "unfortunate". . . . The false minimizings: "I'm going to pop a little IV in your groin," I once said brightly to a half-conscious patient, while standing over her with a six-inch-long quarter-inch-thick intravenous catheter. "The phrase, 'a little cramping,' should have cued me in," said another patient, after an endometrial biopsy in her gynecologist's office. "When they say that, run for the hills."

If using words that are too indirect is one problem, using ones that are too strong can be another. I don't have the best history with this; at the age of four, I was thrown out my preschool for swearing, an illustrious beginning to my academic career.

It was, apparently, a repeated pattern rather than a single incident. My father, among his other faults and virtues, was a man of colorful vocabulary, and apart from the broad spectrum of things that couldn't be said at my grandmother's house, I had not been taught that certain words were unacceptable for use by children, or in polite company. There's a story about me at age two, playing in the sandbox while my father was building something nearby. He hit his thumb hard with a hammer, and before he could recover his voice I helpfully supplied the relevant phrase. "Goddammit! Right, Daddy?"

My mother had been raised in the tradition of swearing substitutes, a "clean" word tacked on behind the opening of a curse. Her father, when provoked, would say "Shhhh . . . ugar!" or Jjjjjjjj . . . iminy cricket!" Phrases out of a 1950s sitcom, which makes sense, since he was parenting in the fifties. By the seventies when she was rearing us, my mother didn't make an issue of what we said and didn't say, until the preschool incident, after which some practical restrictions were put in place. "There are words that some people think are bad to use, so you shouldn't say them or people will get upset," she explained to me. I did not much like to upset people (then as now), so this went over fine.

This pragmatic approach would stay with me. When you don't start out with the core belief that certain words are intrinsically pernicious, it's hard to acquire it later. So an inner-outer disconnect on the subject of swearing was familiar long before I knew the word "professionalism." Still, I was startled to have a few of my patients complain about the "street language" in my first book. After that I began to pay more attention to the language I use in clinic. There, coming out of my expelled-from-preschool mouth, were these funny, squeaky-clean phrases. "Goodness gracious!" I heard myself say. "By golly!"

"Goodness," though a safe alternative to "God," can carried to the point of ludicrousness. "Even in the worst-case scenario," I heard myself saying once to a patient, "suppose, goodness forbid, that the cancer has spread—" "Goodness forbid?" What kind of a phrase is that? It doesn't make any sense. Goodness doesn't forbid things.

I don't use my grandfather's "Sugar!" but I do say, "Shoot." I use a lot of "drat" and "darn." I used to use the word "bastards" with ironic overstatement: "They forgot to validate your parking? Bastards!" I realized this was too strong, so I downgraded it to "rascals," but the effect just isn't the same.

One day a middle-aged woman was describing a car accident she'd just had, in which a semi swerved into her lane. Mustering quick reflexes, she'd thrown on her brakes and pulled over onto the shoulder, just grazing the concrete divider.

"It could have been worse. I've never been so scared—the truck just came out of nowhere!"

"Jeepers creepers!" I said.

She gave me a strange look. "Did you just say, 'jeepers creepers'?"

"I think I did."

"I haven't heard that phrase in twenty years."

"I don't know where it came from."

"You can say, Jesus Christ, if you want. I'm Christian, but I won't be offended."

"Okay, I'll remember that." I laughed. I wondered what my father would have thought of all this. Maybe I'm just doing the same thing I've done all along, trying to supply the words I think are right. "Goddammit! Right, Daddy?"

Another part of my word collection is the words I gather from patients. A charming schizophrenic patient told me the medication I gave him made him "too droggy to drive." I loved "droggy" and quoted it often enough that it slipped into my own parlance. "This medication will not make you droggy," I told another patient, who gave me an alarmed look.

"I'm not exactly anxious," said another, "but, I catastrophize. It's genetic. Everyone in my family catastrophizes." Later I learned that this is a standard term in psychiatric parlance. At the time I thought: so that's what I've been doing all these years!

Many are variants on medical words, some so fitting that I wonder why we don't usually use them. "I get the headache with my period, and then when I stop mensing it gets better." "Mensing," I think, has a much nicer ring than "menstruating." Another person described her family history, "It's strange that my mother had heart trouble, because she wasn't a hypertense person. My father, now, he was hypertense." Like so many fathers, I thought.

Some treasures come courtesy of the transcription department. I dictate my notes on each patient encounter, and occasionally what returns isn't quite what I intended. "She inquires about virtual colonoscopy," I dictated once, referring to the new kind of colon exam done by a CT scan rather than a camera on the end of a tube. The transcribed note said instead, "ritual colonoscopy," which brought to mind a group of intestinal specialists in face paint, dancing and drumming around the fire with their colonoscopes. There is, after all, so much ritual in medicine anyway—the washing of hands, the donning of coats, the elaborate (and critical) choreography of sterile technique—perhaps every colonoscopy is a ritual, in its way.

Another transcription described my suspicion that a patient was having "deferred pain." I had intended "referred pain," which occurs when someone experiences pain along the course of a nerve away from where the true problem is—a pinched nerve in the neck, for instance, causing pain in the arm. "Deferred pain" sounded more psychoanalytic to me, as if this were pain put off from an earlier period in life.

Then there was the patient who, in my transcription, "recently took a trip with Elder Hostile to Paris and had a wonderful time." I had never previously noticed the irony in "hostel" and "hostile" being homonyms, but I smiled at the idea of my patient having a wonderful time with the other hostile elders.

Not least, there are the lost words, the communications that simply aren't meant to be. I was at dinner with a friend when I was paged by a patient, a lovely young Czech woman with a deep accent. I called her from my cell phone on the sidewalk outside the restaurant. It was raining, and the connection was erratic.

"Oh, Emily," she said, "Aemelie"—this was how she pronounced my name—"I am so sorry to be bothering you. It is just, let me tell you what happened. I woke up yesterday and I was noticing that there was a little, what do you say, there was a little bisque behind my ear."

"A bisque?"

"Yes, yes, a bisque, you know. Not a nodule"—or did she say, not a knot?—"but a sort of a bisque."

"Ah."

"It was not very tender, just a little—" Here the cell phone blipped out for a second, and I lost a word. "—you see."

"Is it hard, or soft?"

"Well, it's—it's—" Here I lost another word. "It's just in the area where the ear, well, on the head, you know."

"Hm."

"It's a little swollen, well, I don't know about swollen, but a little frotty. I don't have a headache, but a sort of pressure, no, not a pressure really, you understand?"

"I . . ."

"And just now, the reason I was calling you was that just now I checked and there were two behind my other ear as well."

"Two bisques?" I asked faintly.

"Not exactly, but two little sprots, you know."

It occurred to me at this point that I had not actually understood a single one of the significant words that had been exchanged so far in this conversation. I began searching my brain for things, any kind of thing at all, that can appear behind the ear. Lymph nodes. Moles. Cysts. Pimples.

"It goes right out, kind of like a mole—"

"A mole." Hurrah! A word I recognized.

"No, no, not a mole, a molt." Or did she say, a mold?

I reviewed my list and tried to think if anything on it could be acutely dangerous. It seemed unlikely.

"Is it bleeding?" I asked.

"No, no."

I heard my voice shift into a soothing tone. "It's hard for me to understand quite what it is. I think we should have you come in tomorrow morning, and we'll have a look—"

"Aemelie, I am very worried—I was thinking perhaps I could go in to the emergency room. . . ."

I suddenly realized that this had been the inevitable conclusion all along, that even if I understood about the "bisque" and could explain that it was the safest thing in the world, she would still be worried, and she would need to be seen tonight.

"Yes," I said. "I think that's good. Why don't you go ahead and go in to Emergency."

"And they will call you if you need to know?"

"They will call me if I need to know. . . ."

"Oh, thank you, Aemelie. . . ."

"You are very welcome," I said.

I went back to the table and told my friend about the "bisque."

"Maybe it's a mastoid bone," she suggested brightly, examining the area behind her own ears.

"I have noticed that a fair number of new bones do pop up unexpectedly. Xiphoids are very popular. 'This thing just appeared in my chest last week. Shaped like a triangle. It comes right out of my breastbone.' " I touched my own, the small bone under the sternum that everyone has but most people aren't aware of.

" 'It didn't hurt at first but now I've been pushing on it for three days and it feels a little bruised'?"

"Exactly. Such a natural reaction, but it's hard to keep people from feeling bad once you explain it."

" 'Bisque,' " my friend mused, sipping her soup. "I wonder if you'll ever figure out what word she meant."

I never did.

25. A DOCTOR OR AN ARCHITECT

Communication may be the great joy and challenge of a doctor's work life, but communication at home is no less critical. This takes a different shape depending on whether or not the person you come home to is also a physician.

From the time I started medical school, I swore that I would never date a doctor. This is the kind of idiotic declaration you can delude yourself into believing until the right person actually comes along, at which point you do not say: *You are exactly the person I have been looking and waiting for but it sadly cannot be, because you have dedicated your life to the same passionate and important work to which I have dedicated mine.*

Of course, the chances that the person who comes along will be a doctor are very high, since the people you meet as a doctor in training are mostly patients and other doctors, and patients are out of the dating category. Hence, the truism that female doctors mostly marry doctors. (The corresponding line is that male doctors marry nurses, but few of the men I trained with did, so perhaps there's been a generational shift.) Maybe I was fated for a doctor from the beginning, though I had envisioned an architect. Medical people have some fascination with architecture, perhaps because it seems as intellectual as what we do but more creative, and less likely to page you in the middle of the night. Many of the doctors I know secretly want to be architects, or to marry architects—except at two in the morning, when they want to be baristas, and marry millionaires from Microsoft.

One of my best friends maintains that neither he nor I could date a surgeon, because they work harder than we do, and we couldn't bear

to give up the mantle of work martyrdom. Share it, sure; but to con-
sistently be the one working less hard, to be unable to whine about
work—it wouldn't do. It may be true. In any case, I ended up with another internist. Chris was in my residency class (sharing a name with
my closest friend from residency, to endless confusion), and we had
been good friends since internship, but started dating in our third
year of residency.

There are pros and cons to being with someone inside or outside
medicine. The putative architect would, of course, want to talk about
architecture when he came home. We would have, with no added in-
put, at least two topics of conversation, instead of one; there would be
no danger, as there is now, of talking about nothing but medicine.
There wouldn't have to be rules about when or how much it's okay to
talk about work, and inviolable signals for when to stop. A nonmedical partner gives you a grounding outside of the medical world, a
doorway through which to leave this often too engrossing realm, a
different set of perspectives and priorities. I treasure my nonmedical
friends and family for that, and I imagine it would be a wonderful
thing to have at home.

On the other hand, you can call a medical partner from the hospital at 7 P.M. and say: "The pancreatitis guy went into ARDS." He will
already know when he picks up the phone, from the hour and the
caller ID, that you are in the Intensive Care Unit and that you are not
having a good day. You don't have to explain to him that pancreatitis
means inflammation of the pancreas, or that ARDS is "acute respiratory distress syndrome." More than that, he'll know from just those
two words that a man you are taking care of has just gone from being
sick to being very, very sick, and that you are scared, and that you
don't know how it's going to come out. He'll know the sinking feeling
in your heart, because you care about the guy and you don't know if
you can save him. A sinking feeling also because you're tired, and
you're going to be there late, and the ICU nurses will be calling you at
home all night tonight, and if you're lucky and pull him through, for
several more nights. Since your partner is a doctor you don't have to

defend the second set of concerns against the first; he understands that they're both real, just as he understands that by referring to "the pancreatitis guy" you are not reducing this kind, gentle sixty-year-old to his diagnosis, that you know his wife's name, and his dog's, and his granddaughter's and you're going to try to pull him through for all of them. You don't have to explain any of this, and that's good, because you're too tired to do it, but it helps to be understood. Maybe it's okay, about not being with the architect.

Your doctor knows when to bring you a smoothie at work because you haven't had time to eat and you're now too hypoglycemic and nauseated to eat anything else. He knows to drop it off and kiss you quickly and leave, because you don't have time to chat or energy to be sociable. He understands when you call to say you're going to be late because you're taking care of someone sick, just as you understand when he does. You both learn to arrange coverage for important things, and the rest of the time, to be okay with canceling plans, ordering pizza, and enjoying eating alone with the cats and a book.

Your medical partner knows when to complain and when not to. A patient of mine who's a radiology technician told me a story. She works overnight shifts in the hospital every Tuesday, though she hates staying up and hates being away from her family, because it pays well and brings in money that her family needs. One Tuesday night on the phone her husband said, "You have no idea how hard Tuesday nights are for me, taking care of the kids when you're not here." After a pause she answered, "Honey, I'm sorry, but you said that out loud. It's okay to think it, but don't say it out loud." You and your doctor know when to support and when it's okay to whine.

So I've given up on the architect, and fallen head over heels for the doctor. Eight years in, I'm still head over heels, which seems like a good sign. All the people to whom I swore I'd never do it are kind, and hardly ever tease me.

26. SELF-CONSCIOUSNESS

Occasionally I have to blink to reassure myself that things are real; some experiences seem too odd to have made up. I took care of a woman who was very nice but somewhat difficult—"difficult" meaning, for example, nearly overdosing on sedatives before her appointments because the bus ride on the highway made her so nervous. I thought she was having a stroke, once, before I figured out what was going on. She went to the ER another time for abdominal pain and the police called me because she stole another patient's wallet while she was there.

"What were you thinking?" I asked her later.

"I don't know. I could see it sitting there on the chair beside her bed, and—the impulse just came over me."

I felt that I should scold her, but I didn't have the heart.

"So then I ran off, and I tried to throw it into the bushes, but they caught me almost immediately. I can't believe I did that. Have you ever done something really stupid?"

"I've never stolen anyone's wallet," I said.

She had some trouble with her heart, and I sent her to one of my clinic's cardiologists, who was a terrific physician but had a rather abrupt bedside manner. They got off on the wrong note and got into a yelling match in her first visit, which I heard about later in detail from each of them. She refused to see him again. I set her up with another cardiologist, which worked out fine—until one weekend when she came into the hospital with an irregular heart rhythm, and the first one was on call for cardiology.

Wanting to avoid another scene, I decided to coach her a little about how to behave. "I know you don't really like him, but you're just going to have to put up with him over the weekend. He's a good doctor and really a good guy, so just try to be nice, and stay calm." (*And don't steal his wallet*, I decided not to add.)

Meanwhile, her new cardiologist, who had also heard the story of their screaming fight, decided to coach the covering cardiologist as well. "She doesn't like you, so just try to be really friendly and humor her and get through the weekend without any blowups."

All this well-meant coaching created a charged situation that reminded me of nothing so much as a junior high school date: both the patient and the cardiologist were on eggshells, having much more third-party information than was good for them. After the weekend I got the blow-by-blow from both sides.

"He came in and apologized for being himself," she told me.

"She said it wasn't my fault, I just remind her of her ex-husband," he told me.

From there, apparently, they got into a discussion about relationships.

"I said, 'You're not married?' and he said, 'No one will have me,' which really was pretty endearing, although I'm sure he was just trying to hoodwink me."

They were both pleased, and her health was improving as well; a good weekend, all around. I laughed at all the self-consciousness of each of the players in this tangled web. I tried to remember when I had last given so much thought to an interaction with someone who wasn't seriously ill. As I was thinking about this, I noticed that one of the people on the day's schedule was the man I'd seen with blood in his semen just as I was starting practice. In the intervening years this problem, like so many other often-repeated interactions, had become routine; it would no more occur to me to be embarrassed discussing a man's prostate issues than doing a woman's Pap smear.

Self-consciousness, I realized, was all about the unfamiliar; there was no way to predict what would bring it forth the next time. I hoped there wouldn't be screaming matches or stolen wallets involved.

27. TIME

"We'll see you next month then," my grandmother said on one of our Sunday night calls. I had just made reservations to fly out for a visit. "If we're still here."

After my father died, she started talking more about death. Her conversations were peppered with phrases like "when we go" and "if we're still here." She began to leave little musings on my answering machine—a novelty in itself, since for many years she flatly refused to use the machine, while complaining vociferously about how hard it was to reach me. Around her ninetieth birthday she started leaving short messages in a tenuous tone, never convinced that the recording would work. "This is your grandmother," she would begin, then give a sentence or two, and hang up. She never said good-bye to the machine. "I'm just calling," her whispery voice said one day, "to say that when we go, I want you not to grieve. We had a good life, but we've lived too long."

Then I heard the click, and silence.

In the spring of 2004, her ninety-first year and my grandfather's eighty-ninth, they decided they wanted to make it to November. It would be my grandfather's ninetieth birthday, but their bigger incentive was the national election. At this stage, my grandmother explained, getting to vote against George Bush was as good a reason to live as any.

"The world's going to hell," she said. She always made a guilty face after cursing, a mute apology to the nuns of her Catholic girlhood, but she swore anyway. "It's all very well for us, we'll be dead; but you kids are going to have a mess on your hands. Not that it will help much, but we'll try to get to November and do our part."

They talked about November as if it were a destination, a place rather than a time.

The rhythm of my visits to my grandparents was always much the same. I would fly out on Friday night, swapping my white coat and stethoscope for comfy clothes and an inflatable pillow. I hated the red-eye, residency having given me a deep distaste for sleep deprivation, but it was worth it to have an extra day with them. I was often a little sleepy through the weekend, which suited the lowered energy of their age. Most often I took the cheap JetBlue midnight red-eye, flight 86 nonstop from Seattle to JFK. I arrived bleary in New York at eight on Saturday morning, took the shuttle to the rental car terminal, and drove the few hours across New Jersey to my grandparents' house in Pennsylvania. It was always surreal to find myself in this other world, twelve hours after shutting my office door. The drive was mesmerizingly familiar, the same hillsides wrapped each time in different foliage. I crossed the Delaware River and pulled into my grandparents' long driveway just before lunchtime.

They met me at the door each time, my grandmother with a flurry of kisses on my cheeks, my grandfather with a hug and an attempt to take my suitcase, which I always insisted I could carry. I would go upstairs and wash up, standing at the yellow sink I'd known since childhood, and splashing cold water on my face. Then we would have lunch.

When I was in college, the great luxury that epitomized my visits to my grandparents was food: leaving the bland utilitarianism of the college dining hall and coming to this magical place where everything I put into my mouth was a delight. Now, with equal wonder, I wrapped myself in the luxury of time.

If there was one facet of the medical life I didn't understand before entering it, it was how scarce a resource time would be. My workdays are divided into ten-minute increments; each patient gets a certain number of increments depending on the reason for the appointment: from ten minutes for a cold up to forty for an older patient having a physical. In theory everyone is allotted just the amount of time they need, but, of course, sometimes "a cold" is really "a cold and a rash and a little chest pain," or "a cold and my brother just died, and I wasn't planning to talk to you about depression but I'm not sure I can keep going, feeling like this." Every minute of the day I know exactly what time it is, how much time I am supposed to have left for the patient I'm with, and, sadly often, how many minutes I am behind. Not quite the hardest part of my job but probably the most frustrating is the endlessly imperfect effort to reconcile human beings and their needs to the confines of a schedule. My days are a battle over minutes, a struggle between the needs of the person in front of me and the person waiting in the next room. Meantime, of course, I am trying to make each patient feel like he or she is the only person in the world, like I have all the time we could need and no concerns about anyone else—even while my silent tabulation of minutes continues.

In my grandparents' house, time was at a halt. The light sifting through the curtains was the same as it was when the house was built, in my grandfather's boyhood close to a century ago. The house was full of French furniture and heirlooms from my grandmother's family, some of it hundreds of years old. An hour—six whole ten-minute blocks!—or an afternoon drifted by like so many other afternoons, another speck of dust wafting onto the piano. A calendar in the kitchen marked events: a doctor's appointment, a concert, garbage day—but otherwise the days were much the same. In my regular life, time was like a kitchen timer, wound up and ticking down, a buzzer always about to ring. Here, it drifted lazily, a slow deep river. We floated comfortably from lunch to a nap to a little walk to dinner. We talked. I played the piano. There were no minutes to answer to. I always took off my watch and tucked it into my bag.

My grandmother, never a mincer of words, became downright blunt in her advancing age. Sometimes she would precipitate my visits with a demand: "You'd better come. We're going to die soon, and then you'll feel guilty." Her favorite topic was my failure to have children, an issue on which she wasted neither delicacy nor political correctness. "The world is filling up with stupid people and it's all your fault."

"Mine?" I would ask.

"People like you. People who should have children and don't, so it's left to the stupid ones. No wonder everything is such a mess."

"Ah."

"Besides, later you'll wish you had and then it will be too late."

For my part, I finally learned a lesson in directness that I could have gleaned from her a lifetime before, or, failing that, from my profession ten years sooner. After sitting with so many patients for so many years asking questions about their lives, I wonder how I failed to see that I could do the same with the person whose stories and history I cared about most. For years I had waited for the lucky moments when she would talk about her family, about France, about my father's childhood. Not quite too late, I realized that all that was needed was to ask.

Now there was a new shape to our long, lazy afternoons. We would sit in the living room, my grandmother and I on the old French sofa and my grandfather perched on a chair nearby. She would tell stories, with my grandfather tossing in details and corrections. The pretty gold French clock on the mantel rang a tinkling bell every half hour, but the sound was less a marker of the hours than a link to all the other days and decades in which it had rung. We wandered through World War I and World War II, stories from my grandmother's girlhood ("Well, you know about the time I won the Latin prize at the lycee—No? Ah, there's a story—"), my father's boyhood ("There was the time the boys were playing with the coal shovel in the snow and lost it, and there was a great fuss about whether the furnace would go out . . ."), and family tales from before she was born ("My grandfather's grandfather fled to Belgium during the Revolution, and fathered a child without being married—that was very shocking in those days . . ."). Time was something malleable that we could move through at our leisure. The only constraint on these days with my grandparents was knowing that they wouldn't live forever, and wanting to cling to every moment with them I could.

During one of these visits, I discovered that the familiar stories about me had changed. One afternoon, my grandmother launched into the much-repeated tale of my first visit to the house. "You were about three, and we came to visit your great-grandmother, who lived here then. You wore this lovely dress, you looked just darling—You were not much for wearing dresses then, you know. And you went running off into the garden, and within minutes you were covered in dirt, just covered."

She laughed. I'd heard this story so often I knew not only the words but also her inflections as she spoke them.

"And you know what I did," she went on. "I tossed the dress in the wash, dried it and it was just like new—Never could have seen the difference."

I blinked. This was an entirely new ending. A hundred times I'd heard this story, and it always ended with me dirty and disgraced in my great-grandmother's kitchen.

Later that evening, at dinner, she was trying to feed me the last of the potatoes. Her fixation on getting people to eat had not changed over the years. "Won't you have that final bit? You've always been a big eater," she added. "I remember that time we drove you to Florida—"

This is another tale from the collection, the "little Emily is rude to the waitress" story.

"We got in very late, and we were all hungry; and the hotel restaurant was closed. So we went to this place down the street,

where the service was quite slow. And finally you grabbed the waitress as she went by, tugged on her apron and said: 'Miss, I am *very*
hungry—' "

My grandfather and I laughed on cue.

"It was a good thing too," she added, after a pause. "She was very
slow. Maurice"—the most revered of the old French family patriarchs—
"would have done the same thing."

Another new ending! I stared, amazed. Was history being re-
vised, or had these alternate interpretations been there all along,
waiting for me to grow into them?

I usually went back to Seattle on Monday night, the incoming trip repeated in reverse, from the driveway to the river to New Jersey to New
York. I took the Staten Island Expressway to Brooklyn, and then the
Belt Parkway to JFK, usually around sunset to catch the evening flight.
Curling along the shore, I would feel my chest tighten, the setting sun
on the water so beautiful and sad, a metaphor for the knowledge that I
might never see my grandparents again. Waiting in the familiar Jet-
Blue terminal I wanted to stop the sun before it slipped below the
horizon, to believe that love could do the impossible, could preserve
my family against the ravages of time.

The night invariably fell, and the airplane doors opened. I put my
watch back on and strapped myself into my seat, coming home to my
world of ten-minute intervals and the relentless forward motion of
time.

28. ONE-LINERS

Here's to that wonderful drink, the martini
I can take one or two at the most;
After three I am under the table,
After four I am under the host.

Dorothy Parker supposedly penned this quip, but it was quoted to me with great zest by another sparkly older woman, a patient of mine with a wicked grin. If the deep relationships and touching moments are what make the work I do worthwhile, the funny one-liners (or in this case, four) are the icing on the cake.

Alcohol, for all its perils, seems to inspire a good many of them. "I didn't fall off the wagon, I fell under the wagon," one person said ruefully, describing her alcoholic relapse. Another explained, "I don't think I'm an alcoholic. But my husband is definitely an alcoholic and I try to keep up with him." I expressed my concern, but allowed myself to smile at her phrasing. Yet another described her habits: "I love exercise—but I just, I just don't do it very much." "Why not?" I asked. "Well, it interferes with my drinking."

Exercise is another topic that inspires great lines. "Do you exercise regularly?" I asked someone, and she replied without missing a beat: "I jump to conclusions." Another man, the founder of a company, described his work as a sort of exercise: "I created a train and now I get to run in front of it." A majority of people give the exercise question the non-answer, "Not as much as I should," but a surprising number reply, "I floss my teeth." I hear this maybe twice a week, and despite the apparent nonsequitur, people don't exactly seem to mean it as a joke. It's an offering of one good habit in defense of the absence of another. Dentistry and physical exertion seem to be linked in many people's minds: "The dentist, I hate almost as much as exercise," groaned one, the ultimate put-down.

Others have better experiences. A woman who had with great difficulty achieved a much-wanted pregnancy gushed about her exercise routine. "The yoga has been wonderful! I wonder if that's what got me pregnant? I mean . . . not immaculately or anything. . . ." I smiled, and she blushed.

Some people drew unexpected lessons from their experience. "I was talking to my friend's dad, who started smoking when he was fifteen. He told me about this moment when he was thirty years old and he was running for the bus. He got so short of breath, running for the bus, that he decided then and there that he would never run again."

Exercise, I discovered, can be a dangerous as well as healthy activity. I advised a patient who happened to be a lawyer that she ought to exercise more. She returned a month later announcing that on my recommendation she had gone for a walk in the woods, and had been shot at by a hunter. I wondered whether she could sue me.

Food and weight are another rich subject. "I'm wearing very heavy earrings," said one patient, defending the high result on the scale. Another admitted that she lied about her age and weight to the computer on her elliptical training machine. "Do you think it's going to judge you?" I asked, and she shrugged.

"I seldom eat anything with sugar," said another. "Except the cake. And the chocolate. And some candy in the afternoons." Another explained, "Calcium . . . well . . . I only eat cheese in tacos, and I don't eat that many tacos." I concurred that not eating enough tacos to maintain a full calcium supply was probably a good idea.

Aging is approached by many with great humor. "Growing old ain't for sissies," as Bette Davis said, and as many wonderful patients have reminded me. Although, as another said, "As we used to say in the army, if you're still bitchin', you're okay." Of course, the definition of age can vary widely. A patient of Chris's came in to him complaining about the "emptiness" he experienced with aging. "Emptiness?" "Well, there's just this terrible emptiness that descends on you when you turn thirty." One of my patients rather airily accepted the death of an uncle: "He was old. He had spurs on his feet and stuff. It was time for him to let go." It turned out he was sixty. Other family members fared better: "Mother had a stroke at ninety-five. She's wobbly, but fine." Or another: "Mom's ninety. She's a congenital liar, but I guess that's not a medical condition."

Another woman talked about her plans for her dotage. "My sister asked me, 'When you retire, will you move home to Walla Walla?'—that was where we grew up. I said, 'No.' She said, 'I don't mean just, when you retire, but like, when you're really old, I mean, when you get senile. . . .' I said, 'I'd have to be really senile to move back to Walla Walla.'" I've visited Walla Walla, Washington and thought it was lovely, but to each her own.

One woman was philosophical about her failing health. "You're stuck with the body you have. As my mother always used to say, 'You can't make chicken salad out of chicken shit.'" I confessed I had not learned this particular adage on my own mother's knee. Good health can be inspiring, too. "I'm wonderfully dense," said one older woman, in reference to her excellent bone strength. "So am I, apparently," I said a moment later, after accidentally knocking her chart onto the floor. Yet another patient had no intention of going out easy: "I'm too ornery to die. I'm going to live to a hundred and four and then I'm gonna get shot by a jealous wife."

One of Chris's patients almost lost his chance to live that long, having delayed coming in for chest pain that turned out to be a heart attack. "It wasn't an elephant," he explained. "It was a horse sitting on my chest. I would have called you if it was an elephant."

Gender, relationships, and sex may be the ripest materials of all. A bright seventy-year-old woman came down to my office after her mammogram to announce, "If men had to squish their testicles in that machine, they'd have developed another way!" Another's condemnation of the male sex was more all-encompassing: "I don't hate men, but I just don't find much justification for their being here on earth." Sometimes I hear about relationships that are going unexpectedly well: "I was a rabid feminist, and he was—well, from his point of view women were pretty much just semen receptacles," said one woman, describing her husband of forty years, whom she married three weeks after meeting him. Others are going badly. "A friend told me: Cry in the shower; yell in the car," said someone about the end of a seven-year relationship. "So far, it seems to be working." Then there are those where it's hard to tell. "I realized I really prefer being single. I mean . . . I'm married right now . . . so . . . that's okay, I guess. But if I had a choice, I would be single. I mean, I do have a choice I guess, but. . . ." Or another: "I haven't really smoked in years, but I do still smoke one cigarette per week, on Fridays." Why? "To torment my husband."

Both sex and the lack of it can be good subjects for humor. "Things aren't going so well down there." "Do you still want sex and it doesn't work, or are you not interested in it?" "I'm not *dead*, doc!"

Another woman explained about an unexpected hemorrhage, "When the bleeding started, I thought, 'Oh my god, I'm having another miscarriage.' And then I thought, 'No, wait, I haven't had sex in fourteen years.' "

An eighty-five-year-old, with her husband and son in the room, told me, "At my last exam my gynecologist said, 'Marian, it's time for you to think about having an affair.' I said, 'It's okay with me, but Paul Newman is getting a little old.' "

Others are more practical. "I went to the urologist. The pills didn't work, and they wanted me to use a needle. A hypodermic needle, in my penis! I tried it. There's no sex in the world worth that. I'll take up Parcheesi."

One of my favorite lines ever combined sex with another unexpectedly fertile topic for one-liners, antidepressants. "Okay, I'll go back on the antidepressant. Is that the one with the sexual side effects? You can ride the train but you just can't get to the station. I get carpal tunnel syndrome every time I go on that." It took me a minute to figure out what she meant, and then I coughed to stifle a laugh. She giggled, "I actually made you blush! That's pretty funny."

Another patient complained of a different kind of side effect. "I take that medication for PMS. I wanted to get off it. It doesn't let me be as obsessive as I usually enjoy being. That's depressing; it's like I've lost my biggest hobby." Some people tolerated their medications to humor those around them. "The people at work took up a collection so I could go back on the Prozac." Others felt they had no choice. "My therapist told me, 'Depression is like an ulcer. You do it to yourself, but you can't help it.' "

Doctors and doctoring, of course, bear the brunt of many good lines. "The surgeon came in," one patient told me, "and I said, 'Only two kinds of people walk into a room wearing a mask and carrying a weapon: doctors and bank robbers.' " Some are accidentally funny: "My doctor was on vacation so there was another doctor covering up."

One patient told me she almost killed one of her doctors. "Why?" I asked warily. "No, I don't mean it like that," she said. "Really killed him. I went in and he was examining me and suddenly he started sniffling. Then he said, 'Just a minute,' and he left, and he was gone for like forty-five minutes. And his nurse came in and said, 'Do you have cats?' And I said yes, and she said, 'He's deathly allergic.' Doesn't that seem like something you should tell people? I could have changed clothes or something."

Sometimes the joke was on my own advice. One patient had chronic itching in her ears from a mild external ear infection. "Someone told me to put olive oil in my ears after I swim, so I've been doing that—" she said.

"Actually vinegar can work quite well," I said. "It's acidic, which makes it hard for the bacteria to grow."

"You will have me making salad dressing in my ears!" she declared.

We get a few good one-liners in ourselves. A young woman came in concerned that she might have toenail fungus. "I didn't realize what it was, they just got thick and discolored. But my manicurist said it was probably fungus."

She took off her socks and I studied her toes. "Yup. There's a fungus among us."

This has got to be the oldest joke in the book, but she giggled anyway. Still, she eyed her feet with dismay and some mistrust. People often have this reaction to toenail fungus. They take it personally, as if it only happened to people who were somehow unclean—even though consciously they know better.

"Of course, if you'd had more strength of character this would never have happened," I deadpanned, and she broke into real laughter.

"Are you allowed to say things like that?"

I thought of this in a sadder moment, standing in the hospital at the bedside of a woman who had just died after a long illness. I was talking quietly with her family, when a priest walked in. He had come to check on her, knowing the end was near, but not aware that it had already come. He looked startled for a moment, but quickly regained his composure.

"She's in Heaven now," he said. "So she doesn't need us to do anything. But let's have a blessing, for our own comfort."

We held hands over her body, and he spoke gently. "Eternal rest grant unto your faithful departed servant, O Lord, and let perpetual light shine upon her. Deliver her from every evil and welcome her into the Kingdom of Heaven, which she has waited patiently through all her suffering to attain. May her soul through your mercy be always at rest in peace and love."

They're a lot better at this than we are, I thought. That beats "I'm so sorry for your loss" any day.

"We did the Annointing of the Sick a few days ago," he was saying to her daughter. "The sacrament that used to be called the Last Rites. So she was 'good to go,' if you will." He formed the quotation marks with his fingers, and smiled.

Good to go? Did he just say that? Are you allowed to say things like that? I wondered. Then I thought: of course. If humor can be healing in my field, why not in his?

A final class of favorite lines are those that seem okay at first, until you think about them closely. "Seems like it always gets better before it gets worse," someone said once. Then there are the lines that negate themselves. "I have that, what's it called, nominative aphasia," someone complained, using the term for inability to remember the terms for things. "Anyone who can remember 'nominative aphasia' probably doesn't have nominative aphasia," I pointed out.

Another in this category was simpler. "I used to swear like a son of a bitch."

At that, I couldn't help but smile.

ENDINGS AND BEGINNINGS

29. LETTING GO

"Honey, I'm ready," the blue-eyed, white-haired woman on my examining table said earnestly. "I'm ninety-seven. It's time to let me go."

The first time Celeste Andreas told me this, I believed her. I wrote earnest notes in her record documenting that she was not depressed, that she could make her own decisions, and that she was ready to die. It wasn't a theoretical or distant question; she had myelodysplasia, a progressive inability of the bone marrow to make blood cells, and she needed transfusions to keep her alive.

These she's-made-a-decision-to-let-go notes were invariably followed by admission notes to Intensive Care. A month or so out from a transfusion she would begin to get weak, which she didn't really mind. When it progressed enough to make her short of breath, though, she always changed her mind. Death, it seemed, was acceptable, but the process of dying was a different matter. "Ah, what the heck. One more go-round."

Eventually I started conserving my earnestness, and turned instead to outright wheedling and coddling. Better to talk her into a scheduled outpatient transfusion than turn everything upside down when she got desperate. This was the mode we were in today. "I'm ninety-seven," she repeated.

"Perpetua is ninety-eight." Perpetua was her older sister. They'd competed all their lives and they were still at it. When all else failed, Perpetua was my ace in the hole.

"Well, yes, that's true." She looked up. "Last week her blood count was twenty-seven."

"Well, yours is twenty-nine. You're winning."

She giggled. "Oh, okay then. I'll live out a few more months." She leaned toward me. "How's my boyfriend?" She had a great crush on one of our cardiologists.

"Dr. Philips? Charming as ever."

"Cute as a button. Hasn't changed a bit in thirty years. Is he still married?"

"I don't think so."

"Not divorced?"

She sounded shocked. I backpedaled. "I'm not sure." Actually I was, but Celeste was as Catholic as her name implied, and I didn't particularly want to explore her thoughts on divorce.

"Oh, my goodness. I can't believe it. How could he do a thing like that?"

"How do you know she wasn't the one who did it?" I gave her my most devilish smile.

"But he's so cute . . ." She gave a wistful sigh, smiled, and eased herself off the table. "Okay, fine, I'll live a little longer then, if you insist."

"Thank you. We'll call you when we've got the transfusion arranged."

"All right then." She kissed me good-bye.

We went on like this for about two years. She continued having the transfusions with only a moderate amount of protest. She talked cheerily about her impending journey to Heaven, but didn't seem to be in a great hurry to get there.

"I'm taking a hearing aid with me when I go," she told me once.

"Oh?" I was puzzled. Her hearing had recently been tested, and was just fine.

She pointed significantly upward. "It seems He needs one. I've been asking for a long time for Him to take me, but it appears He doesn't hear too well."

When Perpetua died, soon after her hundredth birthday and Celeste's ninety-ninth, I knew with a sinking heart that it was only a matter of time for Celeste. She continued to accept the transfusions for a few months; she had things to do, arrangements to make. She came in to the ER just once during that time with shortness of breath. It wasn't long after a transfusion, and her blood counts were below normal but not as low as usual, so I was a little surprised. We gave her a unit of blood, and she well enough to go home the next day.

She called me that afternoon. "I just had to talk to you—I needed to explain. I'm sorry, I didn't mean to upset anybody. I didn't mean to have Munchausen's."

"Munchausen's?" I couldn't quite believe my ears. Munchausen's syndrome is a psychiatric disorder in which people inflict injury and illness on themselves to get attention. "Munchausen's?"

"I—I didn't really need that transfusion. I got in a fight with Elise." Elise was her oldest daughter, who helped take care of her. "I was so upset, I just couldn't breathe. I went to the ER and I was sorry right away. I was too embarrassed to admit I just couldn't breathe be-cause I was mad, it wasn't the anemia this time. But I couldn't deceive you, I had to call to confess. I'm so sorry, I didn't mean to trouble any-body. I don't want to be a Munchausen's patient."

"Where did you learn that name?"

"There was an article in the paper once. And just now I thought—oh, my goodness, that's me!"

In residency I had taken care of a patient with Munchausen's who injected her own feces under her skin to cause abscesses which we had to open and drain. I shivered at the memory, and tried not to laugh at Celeste's anxiety.

"My dear, you don't have Munchausen's. I'm sorry you fought

with Elise and that you felt so bad. You were going to need blood soon anyway, and this will delay it for a bit; there's no harm done. Did you patch things up with Elise?"

"Yes."

"Good. Now stop worrying."

Not long after, however, she decided she was done for good. "I've had enough. No more blood." There was a new resolve in her voice, and all my wheedling was for naught. Moreover, she had finally decided to accept hospice care: someone to help at home to ease her through the process of dying, bring medications to suppress her breathlessness, help when she was too weak to move. I realized the decision to let hospice come represented a deeper shift. At last she truly was ready to let go.

I, for my part, had to face the fact that I wasn't really ready to let her go. She was so vibrant, it was hard to imagine her choosing not to live. She was a busybody in the most wonderful sense, constantly engaged with everyone around her. She declared every woman she met beautiful, and every man charming, and she lost no time in demanding the tender details of everyone's life. She offered advice freely, though not always the advice you might expect. Early on she'd extracted the information that I lived with a sweetheart. I worried that this might offend her Catholic sensibilities, but I needn't have.

"Don't marry him," she said. "Until you're sure."

I confessed my surprise at this, and she explained that years ago she had counseled a young friend to marry a man she loved but didn't know well. He later became abusive, and Celeste never again gave advice so lightly. "Better to be cautious. God would understand." She winked.

She was, though, very interested in pairing people off. A part of each visit always went to detailing the romantic comings and goings of her many young friends. She required regular updates on my relationship as well, and after several years of my positive reports, she finally concluded that I should marry him—but only if all went well for another three years.

There was always a glow that lingered in the office after she had been there. How could I be ready to let someone like that go? I set her up, wistfully, with hospice. She came in rarely after that, though we touched base often by phone. She got steadily weaker, but hung on. A few months after she entered hospice, near Christmas, I was surprised to see her name on my schedule.

Her daughter Elise was with her. I had a young medical student with me, so the small room was crowded. Celeste was very pale and more frail than she had been, but she immediately reached out both arms to me for an embrace. "I just came to see you, before I go." After several seconds she released me. "And who's this?" She turned to my student.

"This is Abigail. She's a third-year medical student who's spending afternoons with me for a few months."

"Hello, Abigail," Celeste said seriously. "Learn what you can from Dr. Transue. She's a good one."

Abigail nodded.

"You won't believe what I did," Celeste said to me.

"What did you do?"

"I took all of Perpetua's things. All the photos, and all the newspaper pieces about her death, and all the nice letters that everyone wrote. Also the old photos we had gathered, you know, for the funeral and all. I gathered them all up in a big pile, and you know what I did?"

"Tell me."

"I burned them. One by one, I burned them all. And I said to her—Go. Now you can rest."

"Oh, Celeste—"

"It's not right, you know. To try to make someone stay."

"I know."

She turned to Abigail and studied her carefully. "You're very pretty," she pronounced.

Abigail blushed. "Thank you."

"You have wonderful eyes. They're like my granddaughter's."

"They are," I agreed, having met the whole family during

Celeste's stays in the hospital. All of the women in her family looked twenty years younger than they were, and had stunning eyes.

"And you." She turned back to me. "Three years. Don't forget. I don't think I'll be needing an invitation."

"We'll send one to you somehow."

She turned back to Abigail with a smile. "It's a long story. I haven't the breath to explain. She knows."

"I do," I said. "Celeste . . . have you thought at all about changing your mind?"

"What?"

"Maybe having another transfusion."

"No, dear. None of that. Not even for your wedding. My neighbor wanted me to go to his granddaughter's wedding, but I said no to that, too."

"How's your neighbor?" She'd told me about him; he'd made her dinner every Sunday night in the many years since her husband died.

"Oh—we had a little fight. It was a few weeks ago, and I haven't wanted to call."

"You should call and make it up. You've been friends all these years."

"Maybe. I suppose."

I made a face at her. "I'm letting you have your way about this dying business. The least you can do is promise me you'll call your neighbor."

"Oh, okay." She waggled a finger at me, but she was smiling. "I can never resist you." She sighed. "I didn't really need to come in today. I don't need anything from you. But I wanted to say good-bye."

From the chair in the corner, I could hear Elise's breathing catch. I've joked that I can find a tissue blindfolded from anywhere in my clinic; not breaking eye contact with Celeste, I reached for my box of tissues and handed one to Elise.

"Oh dear. Now I've made Elise cry," Celeste said.

"She's okay." I glanced at Elise, who nodded.

"I wouldn't have come if you were Christ himself—I'll see him soon enough. But I had to see you before I go." She patted my hand lovingly.

"How are the hospice folks doing with you?"

"They're wonderful. The first one, Karen, she's a beautiful girl. She came from Minnesota. And the other one, Nancy. She's got dark hair, she's from Carolina, she has a lovely lilting voice."

"Have you married them off yet?"

"Not quite, I'm working on it. But did I ever tell you about the little nurse from the hospital? The Burmese one? I met her a few times back and she was thinking about having a baby and I told her—*You'll get pregnant. Three months*, I said. The next time I was in for a transfusion, she came running up to me, she couldn't wait to tell me—she was pregnant. It had happened right when I said."

"You're dangerous with your predictions."

"But wait. I went back two months later and—she lost the baby. She miscarried at thirteen weeks."

Celeste's beautiful, bright eyes filled up with tears.

"She'll have another. She'll be okay," I said. "Some things are meant to be, and some things aren't. She'll be all right."

"I felt like I should have known."

"You couldn't have known. All you could do was support her when it happened, which you did."

"You're so sweet. My son fell in love with you." She cocked her head toward Abigail. "He did, you know. But it's all right, I know about her boyfriend. And my son has a wife. So it's okay. He did, though, really."

She turned back to me. "I did want to ask you. Do I need to keep taking all these medicines?"

"Let's see your list." I studied it. "Most of them you can stop, but these two, I think you need. See—these help you feel better when your breathing is hard. And these are to help you sleep, that's important."

"Oh, all right. But it's such an irritation to refill them. Do you know—I know you can't tell me this, you've explained that, and I know that no one knows but God—but could you just give me a sense of how long I'm going to last? Just so I can know how many pills to order?"

My tears blindsided me, though I'd held them at bay so long. Through blurry eyes my instinct for the tissues failed me. Abigail stepped in and pressed a crumpled tissue to my palm.

When I regained my composure, I said, "Let's take it month by month, okay? Refill thirty days at a time."

"I guess that's fine. What about my heart? Every time I get up it just pounds, pounds, pounds."

"Do you know why that is?"

She sighed. "Yes. You explained it, and so did my pretty nurse Nancy, the one from Carolina. I don't have enough of those red corpuscles—"

"Blood," I said. "You don't have enough blood."

"So my heart is working extra hard to try to get the oxygen around."

"Yes."

"Nothing we can do about that."

"We could give you more blood."

"No. No more of that." She shook her head. "It's okay, though. I just stay still, and then I feel all right."

"So the hospice people, besides being pretty, they've been helpful?"

"Oh, yes. They're lovely. That Nancy is very good at explaining. I had lots of questions, about how it would be at the end, you know, and I think she's made it clear." She cleared her throat. "Well, dear, you've been a blessing, you know. Through all of this."

I fought back the tears that were rising again.

"Stop it. It's my choice. I've got people waiting for me on the other side, you know. Fifty-six years my husband and I were married. He's been gone now twenty-five. About time for me to join, I think. Hope he hasn't found a girlfriend up there."

"Celeste—you're right, you get to choose. I respect whatever choice you make. But selfishly, because I'll miss you terribly, just let me ask again—are you quite sure?"

"Yes, dear. I am quite sure." She sighed. "Don't miss me," she added. "There are lots of others out there."

"There's no other *you* out there."

She smiled.

"What are you going to do for Christmas?" I asked.

"I don't want to tell you, you won't like it."

"Tell me anyway."

"I want to be alone, at home." From her corner, Elise sighed audibly. "The kids don't like it," Celeste said. I'd always had to laugh at how she called her offspring, all in their seventies, 'the kids.' "But people tire me out. I know everyone cares and that's nice, but it's exhausting to have them all around. I'd just as soon have a quiet day. Everyone could drop in for a half hour, maybe. Maybe my neighbor could bring a little dinner, since you say we have to make up. I don't think I want to go over there. Too tiring. But he could bring a little something."

She turned to Abigail to explain. "After my husband died, the man next door asked if I would come to dinner. And I—I'd never even had dinner with a man except my husband. So I said no.

"Then on Sunday night he called again, and said, 'I'm alone here. And you're alone there. It just seems silly.'

"So I went. And twenty-five years now he's had me to dinner every Sunday. A four-course meal. He's quite the cook."

"Lucky you," I said.

"He's eighty-three. He's very rich; he'd make someone a good husband." She paused for a second. "He's too old for you," she added.

"Yes, I think a little," I agreed.

"And you've got someone." She giggled and pinched my cheek. "You're a dear. Now, are we done?"

"No, one more thing."

"Yes?"

I took both her hands.

"Careful," she said. "My arthritis."

"I won't break you, I promise. But I need one thing. I need you to promise that if you need me—for anything, any time, any reason, you will call me. If you change your mind, or if you don't, if you're uncomfortable or uncertain about anything, just call me. You have my number. Call."

"Okay."

"You have to promise."

She pursed her wrinkled lips and furrowed her brows. "You're such a bully. Okay. Fine, I promise."

My eyes were wet again and she gently pushed me in the chest. "Don't do that." She turned to Abigail. "Are you married?"

"No," Abigail said. Then shyly, "I do have a boyfriend."

"Well, you be careful. Don't do anything before you're ready. Like this one, here. She has to wait three years."

"I know," I said.

"Three years, not less, not longer. I'll be watching. Okay, then. Give me an arm."

I offered her my elbow and she lifted herself off the exam table. I settled her into her wheelchair and opened the door.

"Bye, dear," she said, waving to my medical assistant. "You take care of yourself."

"You, too, Celeste."

I leaned to kiss her cheek in the hallway and she hugged me firmly, both arms around my neck. "Hey—what's his name?" she whispered.

"Who?"

"You know."

"Chris," I said.

"That's a good name. You can keep him."

"Thanks; I will."

"Come, Elise," she said. Elise wheeled her off down the hallway.

3o. SIMPLE

I'm on call for my own patients during the week, but on the weekends I'm part of a group of doctors who cover for each other. Most weekends I'm off, but every few months or so I have a busy weekend covering for my partners. Each call weekend has its stories, some sweet, some sad. One September weekend in my fourth year of practice, I spent half the weekend at the bedside of a patient who wasn't the sickest of the people I was taking care of, but the most compelling. He was eighty years old, and newly diagnosed with widely dispersed metastases of the lung cancer he thought he'd kicked five years ago.

"It isn't about me," he said. "I'm not afraid to die. It's about my wife."

His wife was seventy-nine and slowly sinking into Alzheimer's. She could no longer dress herself or do simple things around the house, but she was aware enough to know where home was and that she didn't want to leave it. "She won't go anywhere," he said. "And no one else can take my place. So it isn't quite so simple, dying."

I wasn't as busy on call as I sometimes am, so I hung out in his room, chatting with him between answering pages. He had been a teacher, teaching high school math for thirty years to kids in the inner city. He could spin around from the chalkboard and hit a misbehaving kid between the eyes with a piece of chalk—"You could do that kind of thing in those days," he said, laughing. But he fought to keep the troubled students in class and get the gifted ones scholarships to college.

He told me that nobody had listened to these stories in many years, and he fell asleep with me still sitting there. He looked very peaceful.

Later in the weekend he admitted to me that he had had a suicide pact with his wife. "We were both going to off ourselves if either of us got too sick. But she reneged. She softened up as she lost her memory. She wants to stay with her grandchildren."

His tone was resigned, but a little disappointed. At that moment, though, the phone rang, and I could hear his voice go soft. It was his wife, and she was asking for coffee. "You mustn't try to make coffee," he said. "Coffee is too hard. Try tea. Have some tea, remember where the bags are, in the cabinet beside the sink. Beside the sink. Tea."

His voice was unbearably patient and tender, and I slipped out of the room.

Had anyone, I wondered, ever said that dying was simple?

31. OCTOBER

In October, I took another trip to visit my grandparents. My grandmother was complaining more and more often of feeling tired, and of her legs being swollen. Meantime, the much-discussed November election was approaching, and I felt a twinge of dread. If they had been holding on all this time to get to November, what would happen next?

I took the usual Friday night flight, picked up the rental car at the usual counter, set off on the familiar drive. Fall had not yet faded, and the hillsides were a burning glory of color, the air sweet and clear. I had a rare moment of wondering why I had moved out West. How could I have given up the splendor of the Eastern fall?

I pulled into my grandparents' driveway, parked the car, and carried my suitcase to the step. All the rhythms of the trip had been exactly the same as they were every time. But for the first time in my memory, no one came to open the door. I let myself in, set down my suitcase, and called out. "Hello?"

There was no answer. *Their hearing must be getting worse*, I thought. They didn't hear the car pull in, or my voice calling.

But no. They were sitting in the little sunporch, my grandmother perched on the side of the sofa, leaning forward, gasping for air. My grandfather sat beside her, looking helpless and rubbing her back. She was in her nightgown. It was a few minutes before noon.

I have never felt so entirely split in two. I saw her through my doctor's eyes, a very elderly woman in respiratory distress, probably in heart failure. And I saw her as my grandmother, one of the most beloved people in my world, close to dying.

She had been old, or seemed so, all my life—I wouldn't say now that a woman in her sixties was old, but she seemed that way when I was less than ten—and she had moved into advanced age without my quite marking the distinction. She seemed more frail after my father's death than she had before. But somehow her fierceness, the force of her personality, coupled with the fact that she had always been there, a pillar of stability through my entire life, had left me not truly believing that she could really die. Intellectually, of course, I knew that she wouldn't live forever. We had talked and talked about it; but only in that moment, watching her gasping on the sofa, did I grasp it entirely. I was going to lose her. She might be ready, but I wasn't.

My medical self was kneeling in front of her, feeling her rapid pulse, noting her swollen legs.

"Is your breathing worse when you try to lie down?"

She paused for a moment, measuring her privacy against my probing; then, seeming to make a decision, she nodded.

"She hardly ever lies down anymore," my grandfather volunteered. She glared at him as if betrayed.

"Do you ever wake up in the night not being able to breathe?"

She nodded.

"Does it feel better if you sit up?"

She shrugged. "Sometimes I have these, they're like panic attacks."

"Tell me about them."

"Like I'm asleep and then I wake up and I can't breathe. It's very unpleasant."

"Does it get better when you sit up?"

"Yes."

It could have been a case presentation on a medical school exam. *The three classic symptoms of congestive heart failure are edema (swelling of the legs), orthopnea (breathing more comfortably upright), and paroxysmal nocturnal dyspnea (waking in the night with difficulty breathing)*, a good student would have written. But this was real, and it was my grandmother.

"Are you having any pain in your chest?"

"No."

"How long has this been going on?"

"Awhile. I've been coughing a lot—my doctor gave me an antibiotic, and she increased my water pill. But it's not better. Today, a little worse." She was breathless from speaking so many words.

"It sounds like a problem with your heart." I was irritated with myself for not having brought my stethoscope; it would have helped to listen to her lungs.

"I wondered about that."

"Have your doctors used the phrase 'heart failure'?" I knew all about my grandfather's health, but my grandmother had always shied away from giving specifics about hers. What little I knew was only from when she had been in the hospital and too sick to insist on privacy.

She thought for a minute. "Yes. I think I've had that. Something about my heart valves."

I nodded.

"So, what do you think, doctor?" She mustered a momentary, teasing smile.

"I think we need to go to the hospital."

"No hospital, thank you." After a few deep breaths, she pushed herself with great effort to her feet. "Maybe I'll see the doctor Monday.

Now just give me a second, I'll fix lunch." She waved me from the room, forceful and imperious as ever, as if she could banish sickness and age itself with a flick of the wrist.

Over my protests, she made her way to the kitchen. She sat at the table and supervised while my grandfather and I put together lunch, unpacking cheeses, slicing bread, peeling peaches.

We ate slowly, my grandmother pausing between bites to breathe.

"After lunch, we're going to the hospital," I said in my firmest tone.

"I can't."

"Why not?"

"I can't get dressed. My clothes feel too tight against my chest, even a shirt. I can't breathe."

"Just wear a bathrobe."

"I don't have a bathrobe."

"You don't?"

"Just a summer one. Not warm."

I made a mental note to buy her a warm bathrobe. "Just drape your coat over your shoulders."

"I can't go to the hospital in a nightgown and a coat!"

"Of course you can."

She shook her head.

"Trust me on this." I coaxed her into a smile. "The hospital wouldn't care if you showed up naked."

"I don't want to be naked. It's cold." She shook her head but managed a rueful smile. "I suppose you're right."

"I have some expertise in this."

She turned away, looked at the floor, the wall. "I don't want to go." *You have to go. I can't watch you like this.* "I know."

She sighed, and met my eyes again. "You have to die of something," she said simply.

I considered my words carefully. "Yes. We all do. And you don't have to do anything you don't want to do. But, you don't have to suffer like this. They can make you more comfortable."

"Well. Maybe."

There was a long pause. My grandfather was across the table, legs crossed, leaning toward us. He listened intently without speaking. My grandmother smiled ruefully up at him. "Poor Bill."

I reached out absentmindedly and rubbed his foot. "Hey." He smiled at me. "You have big feet," I commented at random, at a loss for words.

"All the Transues do. Even his mother did," my grandmother volunteered, seeming glad of the diversion.

"Really? My father's feet were enormous." I saw her flinch at my use of the past tense. I would try to be more careful.

"Not as big as your grandfather's," was all she said.

"Really?" my grandfather asked.

"You have the biggest feet in the family," she answered.

There was a brief pause.

"We need to go to the hospital," I said.

It was the next morning before I persuaded her to go. She put on a loose dress and we wrapped a coat around her and bundled her into the car. She sat in the backseat so she could stretch her legs out, partway lying down with her head against the car door. We were quiet on the long drive to the hospital, over the rolling Pennsylvania hills with their patchwork of fall foliage. I listened to her breathing, wet and labored but steady. Air in, air out.

It was a strange mix of emotions to be in the emergency room, relief at having made it there, seeing her breathing more comfortably as a slender tube fed oxygen into her nose. But it was terrible to see her in a cot, her dress replaced with a hospital johnnie, looking so very small and old and vulnerable.

The hospital was at once foreign and familiar, a new iteration of an accustomed form. Almost subconsciously, after years of working in different hospitals, I scoped out the place: the size and structure of the ER (bigger than I expected, with an open central work area, curtained bays, no walls), the decorating style (more country-comfort than the sleek-modernist style popular in Seattle, blue and lemon yellow colors, a flowered wallpaper border along the upper edges of the walls). I noted the level of activity (busy, but not frenetic; my grandmother was clearly sick, so we were attended to quickly), the overall tenor (pleasant, professional). I was acutely conscious of my varied roles, wanting to comfort and advocate for her, but not wanting to step on her caretakers' toes or interfere with their work. I didn't have to decide whether to confess that I was a doctor; my grandmother did it for me, to anyone who would listen.

"I'm here because my granddaughter who is a doctor told me that I had to come in."

For the first time, and with a certain wonder, I heard the note of pride in her voice. Maybe she didn't despise doctors quite so much after all?

They gave us a sheaf of forms to fill out. My grandmother was too weak to write and my grandfather's writing had been shaky since his stroke, so I took charge of the forms. I copied numbers from her insurance card into the little marked boxes, wrote what I knew about her medical history and asked her about the rest.

"Surgeries?"

"Just the, what do you call it, hysterectomy."

I didn't know about this, but I tried not to register surprise. "When was that?"

"Years ago."

"Why did you have it? Do you remember how old you were?"

"My uterus was tipped and there was a great deal of bleeding. I was, maybe, forty-five."

I wrote it down. "Any other surgeries?"

"I had a biopsy on my breast once." How could I have not known these things? "The skin cancer on my nose, you know about." She knew precisely what I did and didn't know.

"You were in the hospital the time you had the bleeding. Any other hospitalizations?"

"I was in the hospital for that intestinal bleeding once before, too. The first time was a long time ago. It was before your father was sick, and he came and stayed with me."

She had a list of her medications in her purse, and I copied it carefully onto the form. From the medicines I realized that her doctors must have been treating her heart failure for a long time; she was on a lot of medication for it, at high doses. I wrote down the names and numbers with a sinking stomach.

When the bright, efficient young ER doctor came in to take her history, I tried to stay quiet, not wanting to interfere with either his work or her telling of her story.

"How long have your legs been swollen?" he asked, bending over his clipboard.

"I sprained my ankle as a girl; my right leg has had a tendency to swell up ever since then." I knew that what he wanted was to know how long her legs had been not slightly but seriously swollen, a very different answer. The precise traits that make a wonderful storyteller— every story leading back to another story, a richness of depth and details—can be frustrating in someone giving a medical history. In managing a crisis, you want things simple, cut and dried.

"Are they usually this swollen?" he asked.

"Usually when it's warm they swell, but not the rest of the time."

"So like this, how long have they been this swollen?"

"Like I told you, since I was a girl—"

"The last few weeks," I finally interjected. "The last couple of years they're always a little swollen, but like this, a few weeks." I had bullied this answer out of her the night before.

"You're short of breath?" he asked her.

"Not really." I could see the doctor suppress a snort, since my grandmother was obviously out of breath as she was speaking. *It won't help to pretend you're not sick,* I wanted to whisper in her ear. *Your body's giving you away.* I loved her, though, for trying. Exasperation and affection washed over me together.

"Grandmother . . . you get up to walk to the bathroom, you have to sit and gasp for ten minutes."

She shrugged. The doctor wrote something down.

"Does your chest hurt?"

"No."

I broke in again. "You told me this morning that when you walk up the stairs you get a tight pain in your chest."

She glared at me. "Well that time, I had just run up the stairs and the phone rang and I could hardly talk, it was your cousin Joe on the phone and truly I think he thought I was dying, but it was just that I had just run up the stairs—"

"And you had a pain in your chest then?"

"Well, it's a complicated story. . . ."

Waiting for the first test results, we sat together in her little bay in the emergency room. She wanted water, and another blanket. I pulled aside an aide. "I wonder if I could trouble you—"

"Sure." She brought a cup with ice for the water, and showed me where to get a blanket. "You're a doctor, Mrs. Transue said, in Seattle?"

"Yeah. It's hard being so far away from them, but I get out when I can."

She nodded. "What kind of doctor are you?"

"I'm an internist. You have a really nice ER here."

She smiled. "They redid it a couple of years ago."

"Thanks for your help—" I raised the blanket, and she nodded.

"Let me know if you need anything else," she said.

The ER doctor popped his head into our bay to ask if I wanted to look at her X-rays. Her lower lung fields were patchy with white fluid, her heart enlarged.

"I think there's a small effusion." He pointed, and I nodded.

I hoped I wasn't making him nervous. "We'll give her some more furosemide to get the fluid off, and admit her to the cardiology ward."

There was a glitch. The cardiologist on call was someone my grandparents had seen before—he was the person who had "given my grandfather rat poison, and then electrocuted him" all those years earlier. My grandmother didn't like him. "He's from Pakistan. We went to his office and it was dirty and crammed with people and small children and chickens and goats."

"There were not chickens and goats in the office," I protested. I reminded myself that she was ninety-one and sick and that this was not the moment for a discussion about racial and national bias. *I can't count the number of wonderful Pakistani doctors I've worked with, and you're lucky to have a good cardiologist in this small town, and who are you to criticize anyone for being an immigrant?*

"Well, almost."

"I don't remember any animals," my grandfather said mildly. "And there's nothing wrong with children."

My grandmother sighed loudly. After some back and forth, she agreed to let the cardiologist take care of her, but only if she could see someone else after she was discharged.

This settled, they wheeled her to the cardiology ward. My grandfather and I followed on foot, holding hands on the elevator, and guiding each other through the hallways. The room was like any hospital room. She complained that the bed was uncomfortable and the sheets were scratchy, which were both undoubtedly true. An aide brought her a lunch of tasteless salt-free broth and saltless peas and carrots, and a little bowl of tired-looking grapes. I winced with guilt for all the bland heart-failure diets I have ordered for my patients; necessary, but unpleasant. She ordered me and my grandfather out to lunch. "He won't find anything he likes in the cafeteria," she told me, as if he weren't standing right beside me. "You'll have to take him somewhere, I think there's a little restaurant in the shopping center across the street."

In the restaurant, we ate in near silence, smiling at each other often. "She'll be all right," one of us would remark every few minutes, reassuringly.

"Yes," the other would reply. "She'll be all right."

We stopped at the grocery store to buy her nicer grapes and bananas. "I don't think the good ones have any more salt than the crummy ones," my grandfather pointed out. When we returned a doctor was with her—not her usual internist, but the one covering for the weekend. The disputed cardiologist would be in later. The internist introduced himself, and said he was just leaving; her regular doctor would be in tomorrow. He leaned to check the contents of her urine bag.

"You're peeing well!" he announced brightly, clapping her lower leg in approval. She recoiled.

"Don't touch me there," she said.

"Is it tender?"

"I was shot in that leg when I was a girl, and ever since then I can't stand to be touched there—"

The doctor touched her leg again, ran his hand over the faint scar. My grandmother winced. I took a breath, not sure what I was about to say, but in that moment he waved and slipped out of the room.

She shot me a *you-see-why-I-hate-doctors* look, then gave a tired laugh. "What can you do?" I noticed that she was already breathing a little more comfortably.

"How did you get shot in the leg?"

"You haven't heard that story?"

"Tell me again." My grandfather was unpacking the grapes and bananas; she chided us for getting too many. I could hear the old "yes, but" construction forming: *Bill and Emily brought nice fruit but it was a ridiculous amount.*

When we were each settled with a handful of grapes, my grandfather and I in a chair on either side of the bed, she began. "Well, I was shot by a friend. I was very young, and it was an accident. He was trying to teach me to shoot birds."

"What happened?"

"It was after the war—this is the first war, you know, what you call World War I. He had been an officer, and he had come to know my mother and my grandmother very well. He was married and he had several children, and—this was some time after the war—he became, what is it that you call that? A mental, not a mental disease, but—like what you call depression. Illness. A mental illness. Yes.

"He couldn't work, and eventually the doctor told him that he needed a break away from his family. To recover. He knew us very well, and so—you know our house was big enough—so my mother and grandmother invited him to stay with us, while he recovered. He came to stay with us for quite some time.

"When I was very small I had a sort of a crush on him, I thought that he was very dashing and very handsome. This was somewhat later, but I still liked him very much, and he was kind to me. He needed something to do, for amusement, so they gave him a shotgun. To shoot the birds in the courtyard. He showed me the gun, and he said, would you like to learn to shoot? But it wasn't set up properly and as he handed it to me it went off and fired into my leg."

"My God!"

"There was blood everywhere and it hurt very much. It was a Sunday, and in those days there were no telephones on Sundays, because the operators didn't work then. So you couldn't reach anyone by telephone. My mother wasn't there so my grandmother put me in the carriage and took me to the doctor's house. But there wasn't any electricity on Sundays—this was a very long time ago, eighty years?—so he said, I cannot operate until tomorrow because there are no lights. So she said okay and we went home. If it had been my mother instead of my grandmother—she was a very forceful person—she would have found a way to make him do it, but it was my grandmother and she did not. So I wasn't operated on until the next day, and then he cut out the part of the leg that was hurt and most of the lead—it was lead chicken shot, you know. But there's still some lead in me, maybe. Sometimes there are sharp pains, and I've never been able to stand having anyone touch me there. For a long time it was very painful but not now, but still I can't stand to be touched.

"There was a big scar, of course. It is not such a big deal now, of course, because I am very old and I have scars everywhere. But then I was young and it was very hard. It was not so long after the war, so on the beach—when we were at the beach—people would come and ask me if it was my wound from the war. I was only twelve, when it happened. But no, I had to tell them it had not been that."

"He must have felt terrible."

"What? Oh, yes, he did feel very terrible. And he was already mentally ill. He got a good deal worse."

"I can imagine so." I couldn't help finding this darkly funny. "Did he keep staying with you?"

She frowned with the effort of remembering. "I think not for very long. He went home.

"But after that—they vacationed at the beach, it was a very elegant place, very fancy. He and his family went there every year. And every year I would be invited to go along. I stayed in touch with them—well, until I left."

She turned to my grandfather. "Do you remember him?"

He shook his head. "I remember the story, but not him, I think."

"His mother and his sister were at our wedding."

I asked another question, and we began another story. It was like my other visits, the three of us sitting together while my grandmother told stories and my grandfather and I listened and threw in a few words; only this time we were in the hospital instead of the living room.

In the evening she sent us home, with strict admonitions for me to remind my grandfather to take his pills.

A nurse popped in as we were leaving. "How are you feeling now?"

"I'm cold. My feet are cold."

He brought her a couple of heated blankets, wrapping one around her feet and the other around her shoulders. Swathed in the thick white cloth, she looked a little like a nun in an old-fashioned white habit.

She smiled. "That's very nice." Her smile—a sudden ray of genuine contentment—filled the room. I felt myself relax, and realized I had been coiled up in a spring of tension since the moment I saw her on the sofa, and was only now myself taking a comfortable breath.

At home her absence was a palpable force. My grandfather and I moved about dreamily in the space where she was supposed to be and wasn't. I cooked the steak she had bought, roasted potatoes, constructed salad. It felt like a sacrilege to move around her kitchen, cut with her knives, and fold her napkins without her sharp eyes looking over me. We didn't talk much, my grandfather and I, tired from the effort of worry. I realized how much our conversations tended to run toward her life, her family, rather than his; it was an effort to find something else to talk about. I asked about old friends of theirs I'd known from childhood, the few of their generation who were still living. How were the Detrevilles?

"They're not doing so badly. They've recently moved into a nursing home."

I nodded.

"In some ways they may have a better arrangement than us. I mean, we have our independence, but . . ." He shrugged. "Of course, your grandmother would never accept anything like that. It might be easier to have someone to come in, but . . . your grandmother isn't an easy person to help."

I realized, a little guiltily, that being here with him alone was an opportunity to talk about things she never wanted to discuss. "What are your needs?"

"I don't really need anything. But she's starting to need some help."

I had my doubts about his not needing anything—perhaps all he needed was everything she did? I let it pass. "Like what?"

"Oh, you know. She has trouble getting around. Just doing household things is hard now. Cooking, cleaning up. We do have someone in to clean once a week, but the daily things are hard."

"Have you ever talked about what either of you would do if something happened to the other one?"

"No."

I waited out the silence, and eventually he offered more of an answer.

"I think I would be fine if it were just me. I would be fine by myself, staying in this house. I would make myself breakfast and lunch and I would go to the restaurant up the street for dinner." He shrugged as if there would be nothing more to it than that.

"You really think you would be all right here alone?"

"What? Yes. I think I would manage just fine."

"You wouldn't be too lonely?"

He laughed shortly. "Well, of course I would be lonely. But at my age, you're always lonely." He smiled at me ruefully. "Too many of the people I like are dead."

He laughed and gathered me into a hug, then looked at me pensively.

"I'm sorry for bringing all these things up," I said.

"It's okay, pussycat."

I had brought a pair of down slippers with me as a present for my grandfather. We took them in to her the next morning instead, big puffy green mounds that dwarfed her tiny feet. The effect was comical but she declared her feet to be warm at last. I added properly sized slippers to my mental list of things to get for her.

She looked better. She was breathing more easily, her legs much less swollen though not back to normal. The most dramatic sign of improved health, however, was that she had mustered the strength to complain vociferously. The food was bad, the cheese was tasteless, they brought coffee instead of tea, the bed was terribly uncomfortable, her back hurt, her feet had been cold all night until we brought the slippers, the room was too hot. Every time she went to sleep the nurses woke her up to take her vital signs, and they were always visiting with each other and making noise. "I do not have a good opinion of this place at all," she declared. "I would not trade a night here for two more weeks of living."

"But it's not so much about how long you have as about how you feel while you're doing it—"

"Perhaps I could get some help. Those hospice people who come and give you morphine and get it over with."

I thought of my patient Nick Palmer and his belief that I would come to his house and give him a shot when he wanted to die. Would my grandmother suggest "going to Oregon" next? "I don't think that's exactly what the hospice people do," I said. "But it's true, they could help, it might be a good idea to look into—"

The one bright point was that the cardiologist had come. "Dr. Naeem came and he was not at all as I remembered. I didn't recognize him. He was very well dressed and very pleasant. I don't know if he was the same one at all."

I thought about teasing her about the goats, but decided once again that this was not the time to get into a discussion about her prejudices. I settled for being glad things had gone well.

"But the bed," she continued. "The bed is really terrible. The bed is the most terrible bed I have ever slept on."

At this moment a young nurse entered, with a cheery face and a bright, professional air. "Mrs. Transue, how are you doing?"

"My back hurts. This bed—"

"Yes, I remember," the nurse cut in smoothly. "You told me all about the bed earlier this morning. I wouldn't want to sleep on it, either."

"Many years ago," my grandmother said, "I was in the hospital and there was a hole in the middle of the bed. I kept telling everyone and nobody believed me. And finally my doctor, he was a friend of mine, and I told him: You have to lie on this bed. And he did, and he said, my God, you're right, there's a hole in the bed! And he raised a fuss and within ten minutes they had gotten me a new one."

"Your doctor lay on your bed?" the nurse asked incredulously.

"Yes." My grandmother gave a solemn nod.

"I have never seen anything like that. I would pay to see something like that."

"Well, he did."

"I would get you a new bed, but all of them are exactly like this." She gave a helpless shrug and a sympathetic sigh. My grandmother smiled, charmed.

I envisioned for a moment trying to throw a fit and demand a better bed, hoping to make my grandmother feel as loved and taken care of as she had that other time. But I knew it wouldn't help, that the nurse was almost certainly right that all the beds were equally uncomfortable, and that trying to pull some kind of I'm-a-doctor-and-I-demand-better-care-than-this-for-my-grandmother act would be both completely unfair and counterproductive. I smiled at the nurse and thanked her for her kindness.

"That fabric is terrible to lie on," my grandmother was saying, poking at her sheets.

"We should have brought you your own sheets," I said.

She giggled suddenly. "When I went into the hospital for that hysterectomy, I had my own lace nightgown, and silk sheets! My friend Madeleine brought them for me. That was at Mercy Hospital in Mount Vernon, Ohio—your grandfather was still teaching at Kenyon then—and when the nuns saw those silk sheets, they were so delighted. It was the funniest thing. I thought that nun was going to split open, her smile was so big."

The nurse laughed with the rest of us, then looked businesslike. "Do you have any questions for me right now?" she asked. "I think your doctor will be in a little later to go over your X-rays."

My grandmother turned to me. "I had two X-rays today and two X-rays yesterday. I've never had so many X-rays—"

"The two angles give them a much better sense of what's going on inside," I explained. "And they probably wanted to measure the improvement from yesterday to today."

The nurse glanced at me curiously. "My granddaughter is a doctor," my grandmother announced, and this time there was no mistaking the pride in her voice—warm, simple pride. I'd heard her describe so many other people all these years, and suddenly she was launching into a description of me. "My granddaughter is a doctor in Seattle, she and her partner both are. She's an internist, and she wrote a book, and she teaches, and she plays the piano, and she paints, and she takes beautiful photographs." At the end of this exposition she had to pause to gulp a breath.

The nurse, Mary, looked startled at this barrage, but not as startled as I was. All these things I did, my little accomplishments that she never said anything about—she was proud of all that, all along?

"You wrote a book?" Mary asked.

"Yes," I admitted.

"What's it about?"

"It's about being a resident. Stories from residency."

"My fiancé is a resident," Mary said. "He's in ER."

"Oh dear." I made a face. "Good for him. But that must be hard."

"Oh God, he works all the time. It's crazy. He has a year and a half left."

"Counting days?" I asked.

"I can't wait, I can't stand it. Your—husband is a doctor?" she asked.

"Well, he's not exactly my husband. Just about, but we haven't gotten around to having a wedding. We'll do it sometime."

"You have to wear a dress! Everyone wants to wear a dress. That's why we're getting married."

I wrinkled my nose. "I'm not big on events. Too much planning. And weddings are expensive."

My grandmother was listening intently to this girlish exchange. "You're going to have a wedding someday?" she asked.

"Eventually we will."

"I thought you weren't going to. I think of you as married already."

"You can think of us as married already. We pretty much are."

"But still!" She sounded amazed.

I laughed.

"And children? Maybe children?"

"I don't know. We'll see."

"But maybe! That's not so bad. You shouldn't put it off, you know. You're not so young anymore." She turned to the nurse. "She's pretty accomplished but she's not so young."

I laughed. I knew there had to be a "yes, but" construction in all this somewhere.

The nurse went on to her other patients, and my grandfather and I settled in again on each side of my grandmother's bed.

"It's almost cozy," I said. "All you need is a kitten to curl up in your lap."

She smiled shortly. She had always liked cats; they adopted a stray when I was a teenager, who was allowed to sharpen her claws on the French sofas that we children weren't allowed to touch with our dirty fingers.

"Which relative had the cat who used to sit on his shoulder while he ate?" I asked.

"That was my grandfather. She would sit on his shoulder—just there—while he ate, and if there were any morsels that caught her fancy as he brought them to his mouth, she would lean down and bite them off the fork."

Over the years I had sat at the bedsides of so many patients, wearing my coat and my stethoscope, and carefully gathering their stories. Now here I was once again, sitting at the side of a hospital bed, but without the white coat and listening in a different way. I thought to myself that all those years of learning to ask, learning to remember, would have been worth it for no other reason than this. She asked me questions and I asked her questions and I willed every word seared into my memory for always.

————

Then I had to go.

It was Monday and the minutes were ticking. I had a plane to catch and a full schedule of patients to see on Tuesday. "I'll cancel work, and move my flight—," I'd suggested.

My grandmother shook her head. "Your patients need you," she said. "There's nothing to do but wait here, and you can't stay forever anyway. Best to go home."

"But—"

"We'll be all right. We're ready for whatever happens."

It's okay to go. . . . Can't stay forever. . . . What were we really talking about, my plane flight or her death, the small impending journey or the large one? She smiled her resigned smile and gave her familiar half-shrug. *There it is, what can anyone do?*

I'm not ready, I wanted to say. *You may be ready but I'm not, I can't live without you, I can't let you go. . . .*

I didn't want to cry, because she never did; but I teared up against my will. As we hugged, awkwardly, around her hospital gown and her tubes and her monitors, she was comforting me more than the other way around. "It'll be all right," she said. "You'll see."

"Pussycat, you'll miss your plane," my grandfather said.

I held my grandmother close another minute, breathing in the familiar smell of her face powder and her perfume. I could feel the soft skin of her arms and the tired muscles underneath, the curve of her spine under her gown. "A million thanks, for everything," she whispered.

"I wish I could do something to really help."

"You have."

At this my eyes filled again. "I'm sorry," I said, wiping away my tears. "I've gotten emotional as I get old."

She laughed at my pallid joke. "Keep trying to improve that profession of yours. It makes a difference."

"I don't know."

"I think it does."

"I'll try."

"Call when you get home. To let us know you're safe." Even now, she was taking care of me.

"I will."

"But not until tomorrow, we'll be asleep tonight."

"Okay."

"Safe travels, pussycat," my grandfather said.

Tears blinded me as I walked down the hallway. Waiting at the elevator I barely recognized the aide who had helped me in the ER the day before. She saw my face and looked stricken. "Is she okay?" she whispered.

I wiped my eyes, trying to pull myself together, clearing my throat so I could speak. "She's fine. She's doing great. It's just that I have to leave, and I'm not very good at leaving them."

She nodded. "We'll take good care of her."

"Thank you."

I drove back across the familiar roads to New York, to the airport, everywhere I didn't want to be going. The setting sun lit the red and orange leaves aflame, a million candles burning in vigil on the hillsides.

Suddenly I found the sweetness of it unbearable, the faint smoky smell, the brilliant leaves. How can anyone, I wondered, survive the crushing nostalgia of the Eastern fall? I realized I had grown used to living out West, where the landscape is more wild and less sweet, where nature inspires you to awe but does not make you want to cry.

In no time I was on the Belt Parkway, arcing toward JFK, the sun heartachingly beautiful once again over the water. It was the same story I had just left, told on a different scale, something beautiful and precious and fading. The sun sets. The leaves fall. People die. There will be another dawn, another spring, another birth; but it won't be the same. That's the way the world is, the way life has to be.

I sat in my cushioned airplane seat and watched above the clouds as the last remnants of color faded from the sky. I cried silently against the small, cold windowpane. No matter how much I knew that she was ready to go, that she had lived a longer and healthier life than most people did, and that I'd had her longer than I had any right to ask for, and even though I knew that she was right that I would be okay in the end, still I wasn't ready to let her go. The long miles of the continent passed below the airplane's wings, and I wept quietly for the loss to come.

32. PILLS

The week after I came back from my grandparents' was unusually busy. By Friday I was exhausted, and as I walked in to the room with my twenty-third patient out of twenty-six, I could feel myself running out of steam. She was scheduled for ten minutes for pinkeye.

I couldn't put a face to her name until I walked in. Oh, of course—Gladys. She looked fiftyish but was actually in her seventies, a solid, no-nonsense woman with a gruff manner and a dry sense of humor.

"Hey, doc."

"Hey! Sorry to keep you waiting. . . . What can I help you with?"

"It's the strangest thing. For the last day or two it was kind of tingly around my eye, and then I woke up and it was all red. I don't remember getting bit by anything—"

"Hmm."

"I'm thinking I must have pinkeye. Although it's not so much pink."

I looked at her eye, and no, it wasn't pink. The skin above her eye was red, with fine tiny blisters. The rash extended up the right half of her scalp.

"How long have you had the rash on your forehead?"

"Rash?"

I pulled a mirror from a drawer and handed it to her.

"Well, by damn, you're right. There is a rash on my forehead!"

I set my ophthalmoscope back in its stand and sat down. "You have shingles."

"Really?"

"Yup."

"Well, who'd a thunk my pinkeye would be shingles. . . . I had shingles once before, years ago. It was on my back, on my right shoulder blade. I had pain in my back and the doctor didn't take my shirt off and he said it was a muscle. I went for a massage and rolled on my belly and the masseuse kind of yelped and said, 'Did you know you have shingles?' I went back to the doctor and boy, was he sheepish. He gave me some kind of dope for it."

"Did it make it go away?"

"No, it just helped the pain. You know, dope, the kind of dope that makes you loopy. Some kind of a narcotic or something."

"We have something better now. I don't think you need any dope this time. We'll give you a couple of other things and you'll be fine."

"All right." She nodded briskly. "Hey, that reminds me, that's another thing. You've never given me any pills."

"Pills?" I echoed, surprised. She was usually the type to fight off pills, not ask for them—even when she really needed treatment for something.

"You know, *pills*," she repeated.

"Pills for what?"

"I was talking to my priest. He said, 'You should get some pills.' "

I was still confused. Did he think she was depressed or something?

"He was very frank with me. He sat me down and said, 'Gladys, are you ready to die?' "

Before I could recover enough composure to say anything, she went on. "I said, 'Well, maybe not today, but maybe tomorrow would be good.' " She giggled, and then frowned. "No, but seriously. He said, 'Well, you're at that age where you never know. I'm at that age, too, and if something ever happens, I don't want to be a burden to my family. So I went to my doctor and got some pills, for just in case. You should think about it.' " She looked at me expectantly.

"You're asking me about pills, for in case you get a terminal illness."

"Yes."

"But Gladys, you're as healthy as a horse. There's nothing wrong with you."

"No, not now there isn't. But if I get something, it's more complicated for you to give me pills then. I'd just hold on to them. I'm not going to take them or anything."

"Why are you so concerned about this?"

"I don't want to suffer."

"We have this great thing called hospice, for that." Didn't I just have this conversation with my grandmother?

She sniffed. "I've had friends in hospice. I've known people who spent a year lingering on in hospice. I don't want to linger. I don't want to be debilitated."

Something else occurred to me. "Wait—your *priest* started this conversation with you?"

"Yeah. We were just talking about being prepared."

"A *Catholic* priest?"

"Episcopal."

"Oh."

I closed my eyes and rubbed my temples.

"Gladys—can we have this conversation some other time? Could we maybe just treat your shingles today?"

"Oh, okay." She took the script I was writing. "So I'm supposed to take this stuff, eh?" She looked dubiously at the prescription. "Do I really have to take these? Won't it go away on its own eventually?"

"They'll make it go away faster, and save you a good bit of pain."

"I'll think about it."

"So anxious for some pills and so uninterested in others! I thought you didn't want to suffer?"

She stuck out her tongue at me. "Damn doctors."

"Yeah, we're a troublesome bunch. Try dealing with the damn patients. Feel better, okay?"

"Okay."

She ambled off, and I scurried into the room with my next patient.

33. EMBODIMENT

His doctor signed him out to me for my call weekend. "He has metastatic colon cancer. He's close to the end, and he was admitted for pain control. He'll probably be able to go home next week on a new combination of drugs. But it's a little complicated. His wife died two years ago, also of cancer. He lives with his son, who's schizophrenic and has been having a tough time. Things are a mess at home," his doctor said.

I walked into his room on Saturday morning. "Hi, I'm Dr. Transue. I'm covering this weekend for Dr. Williams."

He nodded. "He works too hard; I'm glad he gets some time off now and again."

"I'm glad, too. But he asked me to look in on you. How are you feeling?"

"Not so bad. The pain specialist adjusted the pills, and I think they're working better."

"That's good." I smiled.

"Where did you go to school?" he asked.

"Dartmouth," I said.

"Back east."

"Yes. But I came to residency here."

"When I die—it won't be long now—I'm giving my body to the University. To the students, for anatomy."

————

I remember, of course, my first cadaver. The first day of anatomy is unforgettable for every doctor, a different experience for each of us, but a world-changing day for all. My first memory is the sweet sickly smell of formaldehyde, which sank through my double-layered gloves and penetrated my fingers, the smell seemingly permanent, inescapable for all the months we worked in the dim basement lab.

Our cadavers were face-down, that first day, and the first thing we dissected was their backs. I remember my first cut, the surprising amount of pressure it took on the scalpel to penetrate the skin, the strange, meaty give as the flesh finally opened. I cut skin rarely now—incise the occasional abscess, biopsy a rash, or remove a cyst. But each time my hands remember that long-ago cut, scalpel against cold skin.

What have I become? I wondered on that day. *What line have I crossed, cutting into a human being, and how will this path change me?* It's hard to remember the weight those questions had, having lived so long on the other side of the line. I can't imagine not being a doctor; it isn't just what I do, it's part of how I see the world. I was afraid then that I would come to see the human body differently, and in a sense I do, although it seems if anything more mystical and magical than before. The more I know the more I am in awe of these amazing structures that move so beautifully through time and space, functioning and malfunctioning, injuring and repairing themselves. Needing a little help, sometimes, to get back on the right track. But each is headed to dust eventually; in my profession you can't escape the realization that every life is an arc, with an eventual end. You realize it the first time you help someone through a life-threatening illness only to lose them to a later, unrelated one. Every save is temporary, in a sense. Once you begin to accept it, this doesn't feel like so terrible. What a miraculous thing it is, this arc of life we each have, however uncertain and temporary. And what a privilege to be able to lengthen or brighten someone's precious slice of time.

I still think a lot about death, though differently than I did all

those years ago. Only rarely, however, do I give much thought to cadavers. Oddly, though, I had recently had another conversation with a
patient about the University's anatomical gift program. She was an at-
tractive young woman, brightly dressed, who worked as a funeral di-
rector. I raised my eyebrows when she first told me her profession,
and she laughed.

"Yeah, everyone does that. But you'd be surprised. Some families
find it comforting, when they're in grief, to deal with a pretty girl, instead of the expected old white guy in a black suit."

"Did you always know you wanted to do this kind of work?"

"I don't know. Yeah, I guess. I was always sort of drawn to it. My dad
used to hunt and I liked to dissect the animals he brought home. I
worked for a taxonomist for a while, but it wasn't what I wanted—I
missed the interaction with people, the human element. So when I went
to college, right away I majored in Bereavement Services."

She liked the work, but not the hours, the call, and the constant
stress of dealing with people who are grieving. In many ways it
sounded like my own complaints about my job. In some ways the re-
wards were similar, too; she got to help people during a hard time, to
ease the process of mourning for the survivors.

She came back in bubbling with excitement over a new job opportunity. There was an opening at the University for someone to
prepare the donated bodies, preserve them, and help with some simple dissections.

"It would be nine to five," she said. "No nights, no call. But the
kind of work I want to do. It would be perfect."

"When will you know?"

"A couple weeks. I did an internship once with the guy who makes
the decision, and I'm lobbying him hard. Jeff Nichols."

"Jeff, the death guy?" I asked.

She frowned, uncertain.

"He works at the county hospital?" I clarified. "With the medical
examiners?"

"Yeah, that's him."

It's state law that when someone dies, a death certificate has to be signed by a physician within twenty-four hours. When you're a resident, this comes up a lot; you're spending a lot of time in the hospital taking care of very sick people, and inevitably, a certain number of them die. Whenever they did, Jeff was there. Not as they died, but the morning after. An unprepossessing man of middle age and middle height, with brownish hair and a clipboard always in hand. You knew your team had lost someone when Jeff appeared, a quiet ghost at the intern's elbow, slipping his clipboard under a wrist: "Sign here."

It was part of the ritual of loss, the understated medical acknowledgment of death. There was something oddly comforting in the existence of Jeff. You might have been up half the night trying to save a patient who finally died, and nobody would say a word about it the next day, as if it had all been a dream—but there was Jeff and his clipboard, declaring that yes, it had been real.

One of the magical things about Jeff was that he always seemed, effortlessly, to know where you were. You could be anywhere on the dozen floors of the hospital but at the appointed moment Jeff was always there, never seeming to be searching for anyone, just appearing at your elbow. I believed I could have been locked in a stall in the ladies' room and Jeff would have slipped his clipboard underneath the door: "Sign here." On the other hand, I was stunned to run into him once at the grocery store; it didn't seem right that the death guy existed outside the hospital, that he shopped and ate. He was a figure of mythic stature, as surely as if he had worn a black cape and carried a scythe.

I hadn't realized that Jeff was in charge of the medical school cadaver program until my patient told me, but I thought about him as I sat talking with the hospital patient with the metastatic colon cancer and the schizophrenic son, who had just told me he was going to donate his body. When this man died maybe Jeff would be the person who was called, and—who knew?—maybe it would be my bubbly young patient who would preserve and prepare his body, so it could become the gift he had chosen to make of it.

For now, on this Saturday morning of my call weekend, here he was, still alive, in front of me. With sad, kind eyes, and the grief of his wife's loss and his illness and his son's. Such sorrow, and still he chose such generosity.

We had a service for our cadavers at the end of anatomy. It was a fairly new idea at the time, though many schools do it now. We invited the families of those who had donated their bodies, to thank them. The service was for the families, and the generous dead, but for us also; a way to try to bridge the gap between the body as object and as person. Many of us had made up stories about our cadavers as we went along, invented lives for them, tried to imagine who they had been. Dissection was at once so intimate and so impersonal. When you have touched someone's pancreas, run your hand down the inner wall of their thorax, pried into all of their cavities and unlocked their bodies' secrets—how could you not feel connected to them in an intimate way? And yet you've never heard their voice or seen them smile. The rare moments when a cadaver asserted its personhood—when you unwrapped a crinkled hand and found nail polish, a shade that she had chosen, perhaps had put there; or, late in the term, when you unwrapped the head and found a face, altered by death and preservation but still expressive—were shocking. This learning tool that you had spent so many hours excavating with your scalpel was a person.

Our memorial service went some ways to answering that jarring dichotomy, but something of it had remained within me until this moment, looking at this man who had chosen to make that gift, whose body would someday be under a student's knife.

"It's all set up," he said. "The papers are done. My wife and I agreed. We both wanted to. To—to give something back. To have something good come out of dying. She passed two years ago."

I sat down on the side of his bed. "No one will ever be able to tell you what a gift that is. It can't be put into words. But still—I want to thank you."

He smiled, and I wished the student who would someday work with his body could see that smile, hear his gravelly, warm voice. "You're welcome," he said.

34. ON THE AIRPLANE

I was flying south and west, from a gray and rainy place to a bright and sunny one. Below me were mountains, craggy peaks covered in snow and glaciers, silver rivulets and alpine lakes weaving between them. As the airplane moved the sun caught each for an instant of blinding brightness, patches of water lifted to the sublime like moments of insight or connection.

It was December, and apart from trips of various lengths to visit family, I had not been on vacation in a year. I hadn't had a chance to set down the weight of my patients' griefs and losses, or my own. But now I was flying away.

Thirty-six hours earlier one of my favorite patients, Paul Hanks, a man in his seventies whom I had diagnosed with esophageal cancer the year before, came into my office complaining of two months' increasing pain in his right upper abdomen. It was worse when he twisted or stretched or hiccupped. Perhaps a muscle strain, he suggested.

"Sprains don't usually get worse over time," I said. I felt his belly. There was a tender, firm spot there that felt like the edge of his liver, but with an irregular contour.

"I was doing some work in the shop," he said. "I might have tweaked it."

"Might have. Let's get a scan of that, just to be sure."

"When?"

It was five o'clock on Thursday afternoon, and the radiology department was closed for the day.

"Tomorrow."

He nodded.

"Let's see, that's Friday. Can he come in anytime?" my medical assistant asked, on the phone with the schedulers.

"Afternoon is better," he offered.

"Morning," I countered. "I'm leaving town for two weeks on Saturday morning, so we'll need to have it read before I go."

"They have an opening at seven-thirty A.M.," my medical assistant reported.

Paul took a quick breath as if to object, then studied my face. "Sure," he agreed, casually. "Where are you going, anyway?"

"Hawaii."

"Good for you. You need a break."

The sinking sensation in my chest was familiar; I had had the same feeling the previous spring, when he first came in. "Sometimes foods just won't go down," he reported. "Lately more and more. I try to swallow something and I have to choke it back up again." He had squinted at me and frowned wryly, as if to say that he knew this wasn't so good.

"Sounds like we should have someone have a look down there," I said. "See what's going on."

The gastroenterologist who looked down with a scope didn't like what he saw: a lumpy, irregular mass in his esophagus. He took biopsies, and I had Paul come back to go over them. The pathology report came in by fax a few minutes before he arrived to discuss it: an aggressive esophageal cancer.

"I have a feeling this isn't going to be good," he said, as I walked into the room.

"It's not," I admitted.

"Okay, let's have it."

"It's cancer. A bad cancer."

He didn't tear up, he just nodded and looked thoughtful. "Here's the thing." He leaned toward me. "I have to get through October."

It was April. "October?"

"I'll be married fifty years October sixth. We've got a party planned. I have dancing to do October sixth, and you've got to get me there." He was completely in earnest.

I did the subtraction. Six months. Statistically, the odds weren't great that he would live that long, but you never know. "Okay," I said. "I have my orders."

"I'm glad you understand," he said.

"I'm sorry for the news," I said.

"I don't envy you this part of your job," he said. "It must be real hard, telling people things like that."

It occurred to me that Nick Palmer had said the same words to me some months earlier, and I gave the same reply. "I'm pretty sure it's easier on my end than yours."

After Paul's surgery I spent hours at his bedside, talking not about the cancer but about everything else. His childhood in the Southwest, his young adulthood, courting his wife half a century earlier. The stories his grandfather used to tell when he was young, how his grandparents had fallen in love when they were just fourteen and run off and lived a year in a camp in the caves, working for ranchers here and there, because their families wouldn't let them be together. Stories about love.

He made it to the anniversary, his October countdown ticking alongside my grandmother's November one. He was still tired from surgery and chemotherapy, but he danced. I was invited but couldn't go; he told me all about it when he saw me afterward. "Thank you," he said seriously.

"I didn't . . ."

"Yes, you did. You made me believe I could get there, and I did. I know it wasn't a given."

Neither of us voiced the implicit other piece, the fact that living to October didn't mean the cancer wasn't coming back. He seemed at peace with it.

Friday morning after his scan, the radiologist on the other side of the phone sounded puzzled. "I don't have his old films for comparison," he said. "So I don't know how much of what I'm seeing is new. There's a ten-centimeter metastasis in his liver. Plus a bunch of smaller ones. And a pleural effusion on the right, and a bunch of little nodules in his lungs. And lymph nodes wrapped around his portal vein. Was all that there before?"

"No," I said. "Thanks."

"I can get the old one for comparison if you want."

"No need. You've already given me my answer."

Sitting on the airplane Saturday morning, watching the ponds and streams catch fire and fade, I thought of Raymond Carver's famous and beautiful poem, "What the Doctor Said."

> *He said it doesn't look good*
> *he said it looks bad in fact real bad*

The patient in the poem had thirty-two spots in his lung; my radiologist said twenty spots or so, in Paul's lungs. Then again, we hadn't scanned his lungs as such, that was just the part visible incidentally on the pictures they were taking of his liver.

I called him on Friday. Usually I try to have an appointment set up beforehand for things like this, giving results that could turn out to be bad. This time there hadn't been a chance, with things happening so quickly. If there isn't an appointment already on the books before I get the result, I'm in a bind. It's terrible to tell someone they have cancer on the phone, but if you call and say, "I need you to come in," you've already given it away and you might as well go ahead from there.

The phone had never felt so heavy, lifted to my ear.

"Hey, Paul, it's Emily Transue." No "doctor" for this role.

"How are you?" he asked.

"Not too bad."

"How am I?"

"That's a tougher one. Do you want to have this conversation on the phone, or do you want to come in and talk?"

"That depends, I guess. Is it bad?"

Plunge. "It isn't great." *It's bad in fact real bad.*

He paused. "Oh. Well, I could come in, I guess. What kind of time have you got?"

"We'll make time for whatever works for you."

"I've got this granddaughter to get. From the airport. We've got her for the weekend, see."

"When's she coming?"

"I should leave in half an hour. Look, let's just talk now, if that's okay."

"Sure."

"Let me go get my wife on the line."

"Hello?" Her voice appeared, and then his. "It's the doctor. She says it's bad."

"How bad?" she asked.

"Give it straight," he said.

"The scan shows something in your liver. It's ten centimeters across, that's about four inches. It wasn't there before."

I paused to let that much sink in.

"That's going to be the cancer, Paul. There's spots in your lungs, too."

"There's not much to do, when it's in the liver," he said. "My brother died of that. I remember."

"Three months from the time they diagnosed it till he was dead," his wife's small voice put in.

"I can't tell you how much time," I said. "We'll talk about options to slow things down, and keep you out of pain. I'll be honest, though— I don't think we're going to be able to lick this."

"I understand."

In a room I would have waited until they spoke next, watched their eyes to see what I should do. On the phone I could only try to glean something from the silence.

"Thanks for not beating around the bush."

I managed a laugh. "I would, if it would help. But it really doesn't."

"It's kind of a shock."

"I know. I. . . . It breaks my heart to have to tell you this."

"I know. Like I told you last time, this is a part of your job I sure don't envy."

"And like I said last time, I'm quite sure it's easier on my end."

I set him up to see his oncologist on Monday. I left the scan on the oncologist's desk, with a long note. I gave Paul my home number, in case he had any questions that night before I left.

"I don't want this to put a damp on your vacation," he said.

"Don't worry about me," I said.

"Thanks, doc," he said.

My ears popped as the plane sank toward the islands. The sun was glinting off an endless ocean. Carver's poem ends:

I may have even thanked him, habit being so strong.

35. A READING

It was the week between Christmas and New Year's. Half the docs in the clinic were on vacation and the rest of us were tearing our hair out trying to get everyone taken care of. An eighty-five-year-old, my partner's patient, was on my schedule for whiplash after a car accident. I'd kept myself running on time all day, which I was proud of. It was all about being efficient, I thought to myself, staying focused on the task at hand.

She was leaning against the exam table as I walked in, not a handsome woman exactly but imposing, with big round yellow glasses and a deeply creased face. She looked me up and down thoughtfully.

"What day and month were you born? Before I decide if I'll talk to you."

I was taken aback. "August," I said. "August nineteenth."

She stroked her chin. "A Leo. Are you an *aggressive* Leo?"

I had no idea how to answer this. "I don't know," I admitted.

"That's too bad." She shook her head, then raised her eyebrows speculatively. "A late Leo, with Virgo rising. So you get a little of the earthy stuff mixed in, more tempered. You like to keep people happy. A mixed blessing in your profession." She nodded sagely. "I'm a tempered Leo, too, on the other side, the Cancer side."

"Ah."

"Give me your hand." She held out hers imperiously, and flipped mine palm-side up, peering at it for a moment before speaking. "Very interesting."

"What's that?"

"Creative. Too creative for this field of yours; what are you doing here?" She shook her head. "Bright, well, I suppose that's a given. Not so good with money, you wouldn't make a businesswoman like me."

"What kind of business are you in?"

"Finance. Well, not anymore. But I was a finance manager, a good finance manager. Not a lot of women in it those days—or really now, for that matter. Corporate accounts mostly. Chain stores, international conglomerates. Made a lot of money. You wouldn't know it from my clothes—better that way. You don't want anyone to know you're rich."

She leaned in again over my palm, traced a line. "You're a little rigid. I bet you don't deal very well with people who do things poorly. Easily frustrated. A perfectionist. True?"

"You can ask my staff."

She touched another line. "An intrinsic shyness." She frowned. "That's unusual for a Leo. Unfortunate—it will keep you from ever becoming a stand-up comic. That's a pity.

"You're interesting. I like your hand. You should come to our parties. We have great parties, me and my daughter. She's in finance, too. She does nonprofits, schools, things like that. Intent apparently on giving back to the world what her mother took from it."

She shrugged. "So, what do you think?"

"I don't think you came in to read my palm."

"No." She shook her head. "Some punk hit me. Driving an enormous SUV, rams right into me from the side. Me going along at half the speed limit like I always do. He's in some great rush and just smashes me from behind. The bastard. Didn't want to give me his insurance or his driver's license but I made him. So what I need you to do, is document that he hurt me. Write it all down. I don't want anything—I don't expect you to fix me. I'll manage. I don't like to take pills. I'm eighty-five years old; I'm not afraid to die, has to happen sometime. But that doesn't mean some bastard can go around just smashing into me, for God's sake.

"I hurt here, and here, and here." She pointed to her neck, her low back, and her knee. "You can poke at me if you want. I trust you. But don't fix. Just write it all down. I suppose you don't have much time."

I looked down at my watch—I had forgotten about time completely. We were already well over schedule. "We have whatever time we need," I said.

36. LONELY

Scheduling, of course, is an unsolvable problem. Fitting patients into time slots implies that it is possible to take people, who are inherently unpredictable—furthermore, sick people, who are even more so—and make an accurate guess as to how much time it will take to set them on the road to being better. It's no wonder that doctors are so often late. My scheduling guidelines, like any physician's, are my best effort at making the impossible equation work, an alchemy of factors that are supposed to combine into the gold of the perfect schedule. We frequently end up with lead, but we keep trying.

There are two special categories of visit that we try to schedule only in the last appointment spot of the day. One is biopsy results; if I might be telling a patient they have cancer I want to have all the time we need, without making anyone else wait. The other is any appointment for Patrick O'Connor, because I can't make him stop talking, and I don't really want to.

Patrick is an Irishman in his seventies. His ruddy complexion belies his lifetime of abstinence from alcohol, imbued in him in childhood by the monks who taught him in school. He fought in two wars for two countries (World War II for Ireland, Korea for the United States), and was seriously injured in both. He was a policeman on two continents over five decades. He is the most charming man I have ever met.

A Patrick O'Connor appointment, whether for a cold or acute chest pain, always begins with a couple of jokes, typically at the expense of the Irish, or the English, or the medical profession. "The doctor says to the woman, 'You're fat!' She says, 'I want a second opinion.' The doctor says, 'Okay, you're also ugly!' " Some of them are long and involved, and require sound effects and gesticulations. They are often off-color, sometimes absurd, and invariably hysterical.

After a few jokes I get an update on the Pumpkin, Patrick's youngest and most beloved granddaughter. She was only two when he first came to me, and I've followed her growth with interest through his adoring eyes. After the Pumpkin report, I may have a chance at hearing something about the reason he came in. He gets through this as quickly as possible, and will sometimes submit to being examined, though he usually uses this time as an excuse to tell more jokes. I have to interrupt him to offer my medical suggestions. Once that's over with, we go on to a discussion of the state of the world, which almost always leads to a story or two or three about his past, which I could sit and listen to forever. I hear battle stories from France and Germany and East Asia. I hear about what it's like to kill a man, and what it's like to be afraid. I hear cop stories from Ireland and Boston and Chicago and Seattle. Stories from his night job as an autopsy assistant—he had young children then, and the doctor let him off when they had to dissect a baby. Stories about the people he met all along the way, who I can imagine were as entranced by him as I am.

At some point I'll pop my head out of the exam room and make sure my staff don't have any questions for me before they go home, since I may be there a long time with Patrick.

On this particular day, the schedule announced he was coming in for back pain. He was sitting on the examining table, looking fit as ever with his military posture and his muscled arms. He seemed comfortable enough, which I took as a good sign about his pain.

The opening joke was about three old Irish women walking down the road with the wind blowing so hard they could barely hear. " 'It's windy!' said the first. 'No, it's Thursday,' said the second. 'Me, too,' said the third. 'Let's go to the pub!' "

Then he told me I was looking well but was too thin, and that I should try a little gluttony. "When I was young we had a very fat priest. This was a time of famine, you know, and we children were often hungry. One day I was playing with my friend in the street and we saw the fat priest coming over the hill. Suddenly it occurred to us: My God, he was a glutton! A mortal sinner among us, and our own priest! Imagine how we felt. We were terrified." He widened his eyes in remembered horror, then laughed heartily. "A glutton. Foolish young lads, we were convinced of the depravity of his soul."

"How's the Pumpkin?"

"She's fine. She's just great. She's learning to play the harp. She has a harp at home, that her mother bought for her. And she went in for her first lesson, with a harpist for the symphony, her and her little friend who's going to learn, too. And the teacher left my Pumpkin alone for a while, there in her house, and you know what she told me? She came into the room, the teacher, quietly on the carpet with no shoes. And she found the Pumpkin standing, facing the wall, and saying: I am going to be the best harpist in the world. I am going to be the best harpist in the world. I am going to be—"

He rocked softly with laughter. "The teacher was worried. This child, all of five years old! But I told her—I think she was just pumping herself up."

He giggled again. "She's fine, a fine young thing. And you? How are you?"

"I'm very well, thanks."

"I was thinking about you the other day. I hope you don't mind. But I wonder sometimes how it's possible for someone to do what you do. To spend days doing this."

"How can you wonder that, having spent as many days as you have spent them?"

"Well, it's different. I've been there, in the madness and the chaos. The heat of it. But you—you spend your days dealing with the residue of people's unbridled enthusiasms, their ill-considered judgments."

I grinned at his phrasing, imagining saying to a patient: *Well, what we're dealing with here is the residue of your unbridled enthusiasms*. But he was serious. "All day you pick up the pieces. All of that lands on you."

"Not all of it." I smiled.

"Still."

"None of this is why you came in," I prompted.

"Ah, so it isn't, I suppose. I pulled my back out on Saturday, I was packing to visit a friend. I had my bag here, on the bed, and my foot was here—" He gestured in demonstration. "Then I did this stupid thing: I reached back into the closet, and with one hand I picked up— it wasn't anything heavy, just a pile of shirts—but . . . There was something about the angle, and as I picked it up something just snapped, and it hurt, under my shoulder blade, just there. So I finished packing and I set off driving, but it just hurt like the dickens. So I called my friend and said I couldn't come, and went on home. The rest of Saturday and Sunday, I lay around on an ice pack, taking aspirin. Afterward it felt much better. Then, well, for the New Year, I had to pay respects. So I went to the old veteran's cemetery, to say hello to Artie Wilson—we fought together in two wars. Then I went to Kenwood for James Peterson and Phil Erics—they were both in Korea but I didn't know them then; we served together on the Force. Then Fremont, for Will James, who was killed in Vietnam.

"By then my back hurt like hell. I didn't mean to overdo it. But there are things a man has to do."

I examined his back, felt the tender bulge of muscle in spasm under his shoulder blade. He admitted that he had gone back to his regular weight-lifting routine on Tuesday, which hadn't helped. He wasn't seriously hurt, and I recommended rest, stretches, and an anti-inflammatory.

"I'll make it a bit longer, then?" he said.

"I do believe so."

"I was talking the other day to my friend Peter Knox—we've known each other for years, he was on the Force. He's not doing so well. He's going to go soon, you see. We were talking, and he was afraid.

"I said, 'Why are you afraid?'

"He said, 'Well, I've never been close to death before.'

"I said, 'Well, I have, two times; and I can tell you there's nothing to be afraid of.'

"It was two times for me; you know this, I've told you those stories. The one time when I was hit and I lost so much blood, and then again when the infection was climbing up my arm and in my blood. I was very close, and it was very quiet, very peaceful. He said, 'Didn't it hurt? You, with a gaping wound in you?' But it didn't. You let go of all that, it's just quiet and peaceful. It went dark. The one time, with the blood, it went all dark, and quiet. The other time there was just a little light, a little fleck of light far away, like they say, at the end of the tunnel. It doesn't hurt. It is lonely, though. I couldn't lie to him about that. It's lonely, there isn't anyone there with you, even if there is someone there. But that's not so bad. We come into this world alone, don't we?—just you and your mother. Maybe in a way she's there, too, in the end. It's lonely, but it's okay to be alone.

"I told him, and he felt better. He wasn't so afraid."

"You were good, to do that for him," I said.

"A man has to help, when he can. It's what we're here for." He took my hand, and looked at me earnestly. "I have to ask you this. Do you believe in God?"

I laughed. "That's an unfair question!"

"Still."

"I don't exactly believe in a man with a white beard sitting on a cloud directing things. I certainly believe there's something more complex than the day-to-day, something deeper and higher. A spiritual purpose, if you will. I don't know if that answers your question, or not."

He squeezed my hand, and whether or not he accepted my answer, I had the sense that he would forgive me.

"I lost a couple of young friends a while back, and after that I had a hard time with God. Tim was thirteen, and for nine months I saw him every day, until the cancer took him. I would go and play tunes on the zither, and he would tell me what he wanted me to play. I played for all the children. He asked me if he could have policemen carry his casket. So when it was time I got two city policemen, and two state policemen, and two marshals, and we carried the casket.

"And Joe, I didn't know Joe quite so long, but he was just seven.

It's hard to believe in a God who would take someone at seven. And make him suffer at it, no less.

"So after that I had a hard time with God. But some while later I was at the University, taking classes in biology. I've told you something about that before, yes? I had this wonderful teacher, he was teaching us about organelles and all those microcellular structures. He said, 'I don't know who the high priestesses of the lipid membrane are, how they let some things through and not others, and just the right ones; or who tells the centromeres and the Golgi complexes what DNA to unwind and what to leave alone. But something. Something does. I hope I have not offended any of you,' he said, 'with my beliefs. But this is how I think it must be.' "

Patrick stared into my face searchingly.

"It's like Thomas Aquinas said. 'For those of you who do not believe in God, look around you.' Look at the animals and the sky and the flowers and the birds. If there are lesser life forms in the desert that lie dormant for years under the sand, and then, when the rains come, they know to come out, grow, put out roots, flower, multiply. . . . Then when it's time, settle into the mud again and wait. . . . If they know that, what force must there be behind all things?"

I nodded. "Such wonder, in the world."

He went on. "And the children. I've always had a terrible weakness for children—it's not just my Pumpkin, you know. The other day I was with a friend at the bus depot in Tacoma, waiting for the bus; and there was a man there. A man who wasn't taking very good care of himself, pretty obese, a scruffy beard. But he had three children with him and it was obvious that he loved them and they loved him. Little one up in his arms, maybe eighteen months, and two more tailing behind, maybe four and five, a boy and a girl. Not well dressed, a little dirty maybe, but they looked healthy, and happy. They were going through the bus depot, and I said to him, 'Having a good day, then?' He smiled and said, 'They love to come through here, look at the people and the busses.'

"I said, 'A fine father, I would be honored to shake your hand.'

I had slipped a twenty out of my wallet in the meantime, quietlike, so my friend who was with me couldn't see me and neither could the children. I slipped it in his palm, and as he shook my hand you could see his face as he felt it. He smiled and said, 'Thank you, sir—'

"Then as I walked away I saw him look at the bill and his eyes light up in surprise."

"I bet the gift of kindness meant as much as the money," I said.

"Maybe. He could buy a little dinner for them with that. Maybe go out to McDonald's. The kids wouldn't be hungry. For that one day he wouldn't have to explain to them what they couldn't have."

He looked at his watch. "It's late, you have to go—"

And I did. Though there were no more clinic patients, I had to go up to the hospital to check on a woman with a failing liver. I wished I could bring Patrick with me, to tell her maybe about the tunnel, and how dying didn't hurt but was lonely. I folded his words in tissue paper in my mind, a gift, a precious piece of wisdom. Whoever Patrick's God was, I thanked Him for sending him to me.

37. MARGARET, PART TWO

A year and a half after her surgery for lung cancer, my patient Margaret—Margaret of the many children, who had the necklace with the bullet that killed her grandson—had a seizure. The CT scan in the Emergency Room showed three glowing spots in her brain: metastases.

Everything happened quickly: the meeting with the oncologist, the neurosurgeon, the radiation oncologist. She was scanned from head to toe, and there was no sign of other metastases. The spots couldn't be approached surgically, but radiation would be painless, and there was a possibility it might cure her.

She went ahead with the radiation. It didn't hurt, but it left her drained and exhausted. "I don't even want to get out of bed," she said. "This is no way to live. You save my life, for what? So I can lie here like a vegetable for twenty years?"

She had made the trip in to clinic because her hip was hurting and I wanted her to have an X-ray. We were talking while we waited for the result.

"I don't think 'vegetable' is a fair word," I countered, wondering for the thousandth time about the grip of this image on our collective imagination. From my grade-school friends asking if my father was a vegetable, to the bright, alert old ladies who respond to my questions about end of life care by declaring they "don't want to be a veggie," we hold on to this odd, anachronistic metaphor. "But no, you're not going to feel like this forever. You're worn out and tired from the radiation. But if the cancer is gone, you'll start to feel better soon. You're not going to feel tired and awful forever."

"And if the cancer's not gone?"

"Then we go from there."

"No more treatment."

"That's fine, if it's what you want, and if it comes to that."

"I don't think it's gone. And I'm so tired. . . . I don't want to stay like this."

"To be honest, if it's not gone, you won't stay like this, either. If it's still there, things will get worse, and then we'll face another set of decisions. But for now, I really want to you to concentrate on the idea that it's gone."

"I don't think it's gone," she repeated. "But I'll play along."

Her X-ray looked fine, except for arthritis. A week later, she fell and shattered the hip. It happened late at night, and she went to surgery the next morning, where the orthopedist pinned everything back together. I ran into him in the hallway afterward. "That area around her hip—I didn't like the look of it, when I got in there," he said, with classic medical understatement. We don't say: *I think it's cancer.* We say: *I don't like the look of that.* "I sent a sample for pathology," he added. "I asked them to send you the report."

"Thanks for the heads-up."

"Sure."

Reports come to my desk in colored folders—blue for labs, radiology, and pathology; green for dictations. Sometimes it seems odd to me that the important ones come in the same format as the trivial, a blue folder containing a normal thyroid result, a slightly elevated cholesterol level, two normal mammogram reports, and the news that Margaret is going to die. Shouldn't it be in its own bright-red envelope—this sheet of paper with its dry pathologic terms: "diffuse infiltration," "high mitotic rate," "poorly differentiated"? The lung cancer had spread to her bones. It was growing fast, changing, becoming more aggressive.

Margaret had been discharged from the hospital in the meantime; she was doing rehab for her hip at the same nursing facility where she had stayed after her lung surgery. I called Jill, Margaret's oldest daughter, and said I wanted to have a family meeting, bring everyone together to talk about the situation and make a long-term plan. We agreed to meet the following evening at the nursing home; Jill would call the rest of the family. I didn't tell her about the pathology report. It seemed wrong not to tell her, even for a day; but it seemed even more wrong to tell her before I told Margaret, and to do anything over the phone. It was better to be there with everyone to talk, to counsel, to provide comfort.

Her children picked seven-thirty as a time they could all come, so I lingered in my office doing paperwork before the meeting. One of my receptionists, working late, poked her head in to vent about office issues. We'd had some trouble with things in the office not running smoothly, and the medical assistant had made a comment earlier in the day that made her feel criticized. This wasn't fair, she pointed out, since she'd been working especially hard to sort it all out. . . .

I spent half an hour soothing ruffled feathers and drying tears, emphasizing the importance of teamwork and mutual respect and everyone doing her part. Meantime, a part of me was thinking: *I'm waiting to go tell someone she's dying. Can't I have a moment of peace to prepare for that?*

When I walked into Margaret's room at the nursing home, two of her daughters were already there. She looked up.

"You're calling this big meeting and you want everyone to be here and that means the news must be really bad."

"Am I not allowed to just get everybody together to talk?"

She gave me a dry look: *Yeah, right.*

I leaned back in my chair and watched them—Margaret with her daughters gathered around her. One was feeding her peaches in small spoonfuls from a jar. She hadn't had much appetite, and everyone was trying hard to make her eat. Another was fluffing up the pillows behind her back, straightening the bedclothes. More came in the minutes that followed. They were all so distinct and yet so much alike. There were differences in age, and in the length and color of their hair, some pale and some brighter in coloring; but all were the same basic shape, with the same pearlike hips and slender waists, and—even more striking—the same gestures and quality of movement. It was fascinating to watch them interact, these daughters and their mother. There was a deep intimacy in the way they touched—all the same flesh—a connectedness that ran deeper than the schisms between them. The rifts, though, were also clearly apparent, some of the women moving together and others to opposite sides of the room, like magnets attracting and repelling. Her sons were quiet islands among the shifting waters.

After a few more minutes everyone was gathered. I left my chair and took the place of privilege, sitting beside her on her bed. I didn't have a script for this, and as I opened my mouth I wasn't certain what I was going to say.

"You know me too well, Margaret."

She grunted with something like amusement. "I'm right, then," she said quietly.

"Yes."

Our eyes met for a moment. Everything I had to say was understood in that glance. She squeezed my hand. "That's all right."

One of the children shifted uncomfortably. "What did she say?"

I took a deep breath. This was my job, after all. I spoke loudly enough for everyone to hear, addressing my words to Margaret, even though she knew what I was about to say. "When the surgeon took out the broken part of your hip, he sent it to the pathologists to look at under the microscope. They found cancer in your hip.

"That means it's spreading around your body, and we're not going to be able to stop it."

There was a long pause while everyone took this in. Margaret's plaintive voice broke the silence.

"Will everyone please let me stop suffering now?"

This was followed by a burst of words from all directions, protests from some, questions from others. It took a moment for everyone to quiet back down.

"Margaret, the question now is really what you want, how you want things to go from here."

"I'd like to just go to sleep and not wake up."

"Well. . . . That's not something I can promise you, although it may be like that at the end. What I can promise you is that we'll keep you from suffering, and help you to be at home if that's where you want to be, and try to make things the way you want them."

"Do I have to eat?" She nodded at the can of peaches, still on the tray beside her.

"You can eat and drink if you want to. But if you don't want to, you don't have to."

"Everyone's been making me."

"I know. But the rules just changed. We were really hoping that you would have a lot of good time left, which made it really important that you keep your strength and your nutrition up. Now we know it will be less time, and we can keep the focus on you being comfortable."

"I'd like everyone to stop hassling me."

"Well . . . there are a few benefits to having incurable cancer. Not many, mind you, but a couple."

She smiled.

"One of them is, you get to do exactly what you want. Nothing else. Another is, we can use all the pain medication we need to keep you comfortable."

"I haven't been very comfortable so far," she said. "If I really get enough medicine, I'm sleepy, and I can't do my therapy, and you all yell at me." Her tone was pointed.

"I'm know," I said. "I'm sorry. Now two things are different. One, we know that a lot of the pain is probably from cancer in your bones, and that's going to take a lot more medicine to control. Two, it doesn't matter if you're too sleepy for physical therapy, because you don't have to do it unless you want to."

"I don't want to."

"Okay."

"And you'll make everyone stop trying to get me to eat and drink?"

"Yes."

"If she doesn't drink, she's going to get kidney failure," said one of her sons from behind me.

Her oldest daughter opened her mouth to interject, and I put up a hand to stop her.

I turned to him. "She's dying," I said, as gently as I could.

His eyes held mine for a very long time. Finally, reluctantly, he nodded.

At the end of the meeting, all the children filed into the hallway and left me alone with Margaret.

"So I was right and you all were wrong, about me getting better," she said.

"I don't think we were wrong to hope. But you know your body better than anybody. And yes, you were right."

"Thanks for not lying to me."

"I told you as soon as I knew."

"I appreciate that."

"I'm sorry."

"I know you are, honey."

I bent to kiss her cheek.

"I love you," she said.

"I love you, too."

Jill was waiting for me in the hallway. "How much time do we have?"

"Not very much, I think. For it to spread so far so fast. . . . And her body is so frail. We never really know, but I think it will be very soon."

"She always wanted to be at home. I always promised I would help her be at home." Her eyes were wet but she kept her voice steady.

"Then we'll get her home."

Margaret went home a few days later. We arranged for a hospital bed to be set up in her living room, and her children took shifts to be with her at all times. She was awake the first day she was at home, smiling and talking with the children and grandchildren, sipping a little water but not taking in much else.

The next day she slipped quietly into unconsciousness. I visited that afternoon, driving to the unfamiliar address. I wish it were possible to make more home visits; it's nice to see people in their own worlds, rather than the artificial setting of the office or hospital. Her house was a pretty lemon-yellow cottage with a beautiful garden. One of her sons was sitting on the porch.

"It's a beautiful day," I said, reaching out a hand.

"Yes." Releasing my hand, he nodded toward the front door. "The others are inside."

A small entry hall opened into the large living room, a lovely open space with a big fireplace and exposed wood beams. Every inch of wall and every piece of furniture was covered in photographs: family pictures, old and new, from her grandparents' generation to her grandchildren's. The ones I knew smiled from the walls at all stages of growth, along with the grandson who had died, and dozens more faces I didn't recognize. Three of her children and two grandchildren were sitting on chairs and sofas, and greeted me as I came in. Everywhere I looked were the smiling faces of her family.

The bed was next to the fireplace; on a table beside it was a tray of scented candles. The room was warm and smelled sweet and spicy.

Margaret was asleep. She gave a contented sigh when I pressed her hand, but didn't open her eyes. I didn't try too hard to wake her.

"She frowned a little when we cleaned her up earlier," came Jill's quiet voice from my elbow. She'd slipped into the room without my noticing. "Otherwise she's mostly slept, but she seems comfortable. She's stopped even needing pain medication. She fades a little more every day, though. I think you were right; I don't think it will be long."

"And you," I said. "Are you okay?"

"I'll be okay. This is what she wanted, to be at home. That's all that matters."

I looked around the room and thought: When the time comes, don't most of us want to go this way? Painlessly, in a beautiful, familiar place, surrounded by those we love.

She died quietly that night.

38. BRIDGE

Every morning begins with quick scan of the schedule, partly to flag the spots where we can squeeze people in, partly just to get a sense of the flavor of the day. Some names get a smile, some a sigh. I like most of my patients; in the final analysis this is why I'm good at what I do—I enjoy people on the whole. But there are a few who are particular favorites, the extra-special tier. Alison was one of those, someone whose name on the list always made me smile in anticipation. She was young, with a wonderful, quirky sense of humor, and an earnest, probing fascination with the world. She was a musician by avocation, though her paychecks came from a marketing job she hated.

I hadn't seen her in a number of months, and was delighted when she appeared on the schedule for a physical. She was basically quite healthy, so we would have a little extra time in the visit to chat and catch up. I was immediately struck that she looked happier, more at peace than she usually did, with some indefinable aura of satisfaction.

"How have you been?" I asked.

"Good," she said. "I. . . ." She seemed about to go on, then paused. "Well, actually, kind of a lot has happened since I last saw you."

"Tell me about it."

"I quit my job," she began.

"Congratulations!" It was a funny thing to say, but she had talked often about how much she detested her work.

"And I'm going to Oberlin next year."

"Wow! You are?"

"Yes. Yes," she repeated. "I had to. Did I tell you? No, I haven't been here since then. It's been a really strange time. Did I tell you I saw someone commit suicide?"

"Goodness! No."

"It was in September. I was running on the trail under the Aurora Bridge and suddenly—there was this thing falling out of the sky. This shape. It landed in the water, and then, after a while, it floated back up. It was a man. Then I realized there were people standing up on top of the bridge, waving. I jumped in the water, of course, and swam out to him. But I had been running so I was tired and I couldn't swim very fast. He was a big guy, and he was heavy, and . . . well, he was dead." She took a breath. "And it was gross.

"Then the police came, and they pulled him out, and they pulled me out. And, well, they yelled at me."

Her eyes filled with tears, and she brushed them away impatiently. "I'm sorry, it just—it wasn't what I needed. Anyway. Well, and the grossest thing was that people didn't even try to help. I mean, all these people on boats and everything, just—standing there watching."

I nodded.

"And here it was this pretty day, the sun and everything, and the birds were still singing, and he was—in the water, dead."

She stopped.

"Oh, Alison, I'm so sorry—"

She shook her head. "I can't explain it really."

"I know a little bit about that feeling," I said. "I mean—I've never watched anybody commit suicide. But I've seen a lot of people die. It happens, in my profession, obviously. And that feeling of—this momentous thing just happened. Someone died, someone's life is over—and it seems like everything should just stop. And then the birds are still singing. I know that feeling."

She nodded. "Nothing like that had ever happened to me before." She shrugged. "So the next day I went into work and it just wasn't right, and I quit my job. The next day I started looking at graduate schools. I mean—I'm sick of everybody telling me that 'music isn't a viable profession.' And—life is short. And I don't want to end up on a bridge."

"Alison. . . ."

"I still don't know what to make of it all. Just that my life changed. Right like that." She shrugged, and then grinned. "And Oberlin worked out."

We did her physical, and I offered her a referral to a counselor to talk more about the suicide. She said she'd think about it. Talking never hurts. On the other hand I wasn't convinced that a counselor—or I—could make any better sense out of it than she already had.

39. JANUARY

My grandmother died the way she had always hoped to die, quietly, at home. When my grandfather got up to take his shower, she was sleeping. By the time he finished, she was gone.

It was early on a Monday morning in January. On the phone the night before, she'd sounded tired. Her doctor had given her a new pill for anxiety; the difficulty of her breathing had begun to frighten her. A great-niece who lived nearby was staying with them for a few nights, helping out. I had a flight booked to fly in five days later. "We'll see you soon," was the last thing she said to me, and "I love you."

I was in Idaho for a conference with Chris, and the news came in an e-mail from my uncle just as we set out for home. She would have been horrified by this, having always rejected the computer as too impersonal a means of contact. Letters, yes; the telephone maybe; but e-mail, no. I called my grandfather. His voice sounded small and faint on the phone, a shadow of itself. The Neptune Society was on their way, he said, to take her body to be cremated. They'd signed up for that, he said. "I'm not sure quite how it works. We've been signed up a long time but we never used it before."

"No," I said. "Of course you didn't."

"It was a good death," he said, almost wistfully. "Just the right kind." It was the niece who'd found her, checking in while my grandfather was showering. She'd died without waking, without making a sound. "It was just what she wanted. What I would want."

"I'm glad," I said, my voice breaking.

"You'll still come, this week?" he asked.

"Of course."

"We would like that."

"I'm glad."

He paused. "I guess I can't say 'we' anymore."

"I think you can say 'we' forever if you want to."

"I would like it if you came," he said, the singular sounding awkward and oddly formal on his tongue.

It was a cold, bright morning in Idaho, the sun glinting on the snow from a storm the night before. It had been a heavy fall, and every rooftop and fencepost was coated with a rounded mound of white. The snow erased all sound, all color, all warmth. The hills and fields and brooks were reduced to a seamless swath of undulating white. We drove through a glinting moonscape, the road its only feature, a fine layer of icy dust drifting and shimmering across the pavement. Chris drove and I cried, staring at the snow, the brightness of the sun painful in my salty eyes. I wondered if there could be a clearer image of death: hurtling through a perfectly white, perfectly soundless space.

She was gone. If my father's death had felt like the silencing of a constant hum of sadness and worry that I had lived with so long as not to hear, my grandmother's felt like the silencing of music, the end of a symphony. She had been part of my life since before memory or consciousness; as long as I had had a self I had a grandmother, weaving stories that connected me to a place and a time before. It was inconceivable to lose her; her narrative was such a part of my own that I wasn't sure I would recognize my story, my life, without her in it.

In the weeks and months before she died, she said over and over again that she didn't want anyone to grieve when she was gone. "You have to promise," she said. "I've lived long enough, I don't want anybody being sad."

At first, I laughed at this, but over time, realizing that she was serious, I confessed. "I don't think I can promise that."

"Why not?"

"Just because you're ready to go, doesn't mean I won't be sad. I won't resent your going, I won't be angry. But you can't ask me not to miss you."

She considered this gravely. "All right," she said at last. "I guess that's fair."

"Thank you," I said.

"I lost my grandmother, what was it? Close to seventy years ago. I loved her very much, and I think about her, and I miss her still."

"There you are." I smiled through the catch in my throat. "I'll miss you till I'm ninety-two."

Locked away at home, I have a list of my patients who have died. There were too many in residency to count, so the list begins in practice. I started it after I realized I had forgotten someone's name. She was a woman who died not too long after I started my practice. She'd been a teacher and a church deacon, and she had two wonderful daughters. She loved Christmas and Christmas things, had a basement full of decorations and lights and kitchy Christmas memorabilia. Necrotizing fasciitis took her, one of the kinds of "flesh-eating bacteria" you read about in the news, a complication in her case of diabetes. Her husband had died suddenly during minor surgery around the same time she became ill. When it became clear that she was failing and wouldn't make it through the fall, her daughters decided to have Christmas early. They decorated the house and put up all the lights and ornaments, and took her home with hospice care. After she died her daughters brought me a crystal snowflake ornament, which hangs in the window in my office to this day, casting prisms. It's always when you feel that you failed someone that they feel you did the most. I wept when she died, partly from the guilt you can't help feeling when someone you are caring for dies, but mostly from the ache of simply missing her.

After that terrible moment when I couldn't think of her name (Deborah; I thought of it a little later, Deborah Johnson), I sat down and started the list. I couldn't lose sight of her, or little Michael Anderson who taught art classes to the adoring old ladies at the nursing home, or brave Nick Palmer, or Liz Williams, who was too young to have cancer eat her alive. It's sort of a poem, the list, each name the key to a story. A sad little poem that no one but me can understand.

Professional deaths, of course, are different from personal ones. Or are they? You love people and lose them, either way. The love is more or less deep, the way of loss is easier or harder. But it's not so different. My heart bleeds for the little poem of lost names.

After my grandmother died I took out the list, not knowing at first quite why I did so, then realizing it had become part of the ritual of loss for me: a way of marking and honoring, even in so small a gesture as the writing of a name. I added hers. Then I went back and added my father's name as well. I read through the list slowly, thinking for a long time about each name, and I realized that each death had shared that sense of something going quiet. A voice I would never again hear, a presence fading into stillness and silence. It was unbearably sad, even though I knew that there would be other voices, other melodies.

Then, listening through the silence, I realized I could still hear the music, my grandmother's, and, yes, my father's, too, and all the people whose stories had brushed against mine and who had shared pieces of their lives with me—those who were dead and those who were still alive. For an instant I glimpsed what my grandmother had meant about not grieving. I had been wrong: those voices, those people weren't lost completely, it was just that in grief I had been unable to hear what in healing I would begin to hear again.

I put away the list, and got a fresh sheet of paper. My grandfather had asked me to write my grandmother's obituary. For ninety years she had been telling stories, and now I was responsible for creating one last narrative, one last summation of her life. It didn't matter that this little version would be necessarily and wholly incomplete. Her story was still alive, it would go on—through me, through everyone else who loved and knew her. And so would each of those other stories, those other lives.

I looked at the white page and began to write.

40. EPILOGUE: KALEIDOCYCLES

JetBlue flight 86 still takes me to New York, and I still take the train to the rental car terminal, and drive my rental car across New Jersey to Pennsylvania, and turn in the familiar driveway to my grandparents' house. My grandfather meets me at the door, his steps a little slower each time but his arms just as wide.

"Hey, pussycat."

At the simple ceremony where we buried my grandmother's ashes, my grandfather spoke a few words in halting French. "Elle etait ma vie," he said. *She was my life.* "Et sans lui je suis perdu." *And without her I am lost.*

I think about the words "loss" and "lost," interwoven but distinct; the challenge of not becoming lost in one's losses. I read again my little poem of the names of the dead: *Liz Williams, Nick Palmer, Margaret Wilson, Paul Hanks, Celeste Andreas.* . . . There is sorrow in each name, and great joy in having known them all. I think about my patient Alison, who saw the man commit suicide, his death becoming for her a strange kind of gift; and how the tragedy of Ellie's husband's death had roused her from her long twilight silence. I talk every day to people who smile through tears in describing their lost loved ones, their own lives building on the foundations of those who are no longer here.

My grandfather has been lonely since my grandmother's death, of course. In some ways he is waiting quietly for his own, hoping that it will be, as he often points out, as good an end as hers was. Yet, in star-tling ways, he has also blossomed. I was surprised when he suggested, before she died, that he might stay in their house alone. During my visit just after her death, he reiterated this intent.

"I think I'll stay here, for a while anyway. Our lives were here. It's hard to imagine being anywhere else."

With some trepidation, I encouraged him to stay. It was a big house in a rural place; the only relatives close by were my grandfa-ther's nephew and his wife, who were kind and helpful but not young (I smile to find myself using my grandmother's "yes, but" construc-tion), and had health problems of their own. His children and grand-children were scattered, glad to help but busy with our own lives. He was shaky since the stroke, and occasionally forgetful; how would he manage all the complications of daily life, pay the bills, do the taxes? There was so much that she had done, all those years—all the cooking, all the tending of the house.

"We already have someone to clean the house," he pointed out. "And someone to do the taxes. I can go to the diner for dinner, and bring back leftovers. They always give you too much; one lasagna will last me three days. Although who knows, maybe I'll learn to cook.

"I'm a bit looking forward to it," he added, an ever-so-slight gleam in his eye. "I've not really been allowed to use the kitchen all these years, and I think I might make a good go of it."

While my grandfather was gingerly rebuilding a life on his own, I was back at work. I see fewer new patients now than when I was first in practice, but every week there are still a handful. "It's so nice to meet you. Tell me what brings you here today." New lives brush against mine, and new stories evolve for the people I already know. Like my father's twisting Escher kaleidocycles, my patients' lives unfold and refold into patterns both new and familiar. People get sick, and get better, and sometimes get sick again. There are marriages and divorces, times of depression and euphoria, tears and laughter. My office continues to be well stocked with tissues.

The poet Donald Hall came back to give another reading in Seattle. I thought of my conversation with Liz Williams about his poetry and his late wife Jane Kenyon's. "Seattle's a good place for poetry and cancer," Liz had said. I went to the reading, wishing she were still alive to be there with me.

He spoke beautifully, and there was not a dry eye in the room. Afterward, a woman stood up to ask a question.

"I came here because I read in the paper that you are an expert in grief," she said.

"I'm not an expert," he said. "I'm an elegist."

She went on. "My son died in a car accident when he was twenty-nine. Two weeks later, on my birthday, my mother died." She went on. She listed brothers and uncles and cousins and friends. The air in the room began to feel awkward, and people shifted in their chairs. The litany continued. I looked around to see if anyone from the bookstore would stop this, and saw other eyes seeking the same answer.

Finally she finished. "So what I want to know is, what do you have to say to that? What do you have to console me?"

Every breath in the room was held.

"No one can console you," he said simply. He seemed about to say more, then turned up his palms as if to say that there was nothing else to add. "What I do is share the things I've felt."

None of us can do more than that, I realized.

My grandfather tells me stories, and in some ways I know him better since my grandmother died. I asked him once what the best things about his life were, looking back from the perspective of nine decades' wisdom. I suppose I expected a flattering answer, like "having grandchildren."

He thought about the question carefully. "The best thing," he said at last, "is when you discover something, like a new concept in mathematics, that no one has ever discovered before.

"That," he added, with great seriousness, "and girls."

He smiled impishly.

I hike in the mountains around Seattle with Chris, and often I swim in the icy alpine lakes, thinking of my grandmother. I think of my father, too; but now, instead of the moment when he asked if I had ever swum in the ocean, I remember how he picked me up and carried me when I fell and cut my head open on the rocks. I touch the scar on my forehead. It will always be there, part of who I am, and yet it's healed; I know that losing him will someday be the same.

I still jog in the early mornings in my neighborhood, the same route where a nurse once saw me running and mentioned it to the wife of my patient in the hospital. Occasionally I'll see someone I take care of on my run and wave, always a bit embarrassed to be seen in jogging clothes and with dirty hair.

One day I was running through a park near my house and sat down to rest on a bench. The glint of a brass plaque on the seat caught my eye, and I leaned down to read it. "In loving memory of Margaret Wilson." It was my patient Margaret, who had died of lung cancer.

I sat on the bench and looked around at the park, the arching canopy of trees, a child's lost soccer ball. A bird chirped in a bush nearby, and another answered. The abundance of life was all around, moving forward, but touched with her memory. I could feel her presence as clearly in the green grass and the light breeze as I had in the room where she took her last breaths. The kaleidocycle turned and took a new shape. She would have approved.

The meals my grandfather has learned to cook are not fancy ones, he's quick to say: a little steak and a little vegetable and a potato. He gave up ice cream years ago, having mild diabetes, but he's taken it back up again, a scoop for dessert. "Blood sugar be damned," he said, pausing to let me react. I hoped my giggle didn't disappoint him.

"I think at ninety-one you've earned your right to ice cream," I replied.

He's gone through the old papers in the house, and when I call on Sunday nights he tells me stories about old friends, or girlfriends from long ago.

He's lonely, of course. Lonely without her, and without all the connections she had so carefully cultivated. The river of letters that had always flowed into their house slowed to a trickle after she died.

"Trouble is, pussycat," he confided to me wistfully, "I'm afraid most people think I'm dead."

I had to acknowledge that this might be true. But then he brightened. "Still, it's not so dreadful. I don't feel bad, and I have a reasonably good time. . . ." He reads, he reminisces, he flirts with the salesgirls in the local shops. He cooks his meals, each Sunday describing to me with shy pride what he made for dinner. It's a note I haven't heard in his voice before—a sense of accomplishment, a simple joy in learning something new.

No one is as surprised by this as he is. At the very end of a long life, and in the shadow of the greatest loss he will ever suffer, he's found the oldest, simplest joy of all—the pleasure of discovery. Still struggling with my own grief, and trying to help many of my patients through theirs, I watch his simple pleasure in his days, and try to learn from it. His world has ended: "She was my life," as he said, and she is gone. But with the incomparable resilience of the human spirit, he picked himself up, and started on a new journey down a new path.